www.wadsworth.com

www.wadsworth.com is the World Wide Web site for Thomson Wadsworth and is your direct source to dozens of online resources.

At *www.wadsworth.com* you can find out about supplements, demonstration software, and student resources. You can also send email to many of our authors and preview new publications and exciting new technologies.

www.wadsworth.com
Changing the way the world learns®

Current Perspectives
Readings on Complementary Medicine
and Diversity from InfoTrac® College Edition

ERIN STRAHAN
Wilfrid Laurier University, Brantford Campus

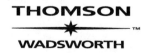

THOMSON
™
WADSWORTH

Australia • Brazil • Canada • Mexico • Singapore • Spain
United Kingdom • United States

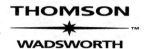

THOMSON
WADSWORTH

Current Perspectives: Readings on Complementary Medicine
and Diversity from InfoTrac® College Edition
Erin Strahan

Acquisitions Editor: *Michele Sordi*
Assistant Editor: *Jennifer Alexander*
Editorial Assistant: *Jana Davis*
Technology Project Manager: *Adrian Paz*
Marketing Manager: *Caroline Croley*
Marketing Assistant: *Natasha Coats*
Marketing Communications Manager: *Linda Yip*
Project Manager, Editorial Production: *Samen Iqbal*
Creative Director: *Rob Hugel*

Print Buyer: *Linda Hsu*
Permissions Editor: *Bob Kauser*
Production Service: *Ruchika Vij, Interactive Composition Corporation*
Cover Designer: *Larry Didona*
Cover Image: *Photolibrary.com/Photonica*
Cover Printer: *Thomson West*
Compositor: *Interactive Composition Corporation*
Printer: *Thomson West*

Library of Congress Control Number:
2006927245

ISBN 0-495-13020-6

For more information about our products,
contact us at:
Thomson Learning Academic Resource Center
1-800-423-0563

For permission to use material from this text or product, submit a request online at
http://www.thomsonrights.com.
Any additional questions about permissions can be submitted by e-mail to
thomsonrights@thomson.com.

Contents

1

The Value of Positive Emotions

The Emerging Science of Positive Psychology Is Coming to Understand Why It's Good to Feel Good

Barbara L. Fredrickson

B ack in the 1930s some young Catholic nuns were asked to write short, personal essays about their lives. They described edifying events in their childhood, the schools they attended, their religious experiences and the influences that led them to the convent. Although the essays may have been initially used to assess each nun's career path, the documents were eventually archived and largely forgotten. More than 60 years later the nuns' writings surfaced again when three psychologists at the University of Kentucky reviewed the essays as part of a larger study on aging and Alzheimer's disease. Deborah Danner, David Snowdon and Wallace Friesen read the nun's biographical sketches and scored them for positive emotional content, recording instances of happiness, interest, love and hope. What they found was remarkable: The nuns who expressed the most positive emotions lived up to 10 years longer than those who expressed the fewest. This gain in life expectancy is considerably larger than the gain achieved by those who quit smoking.

The nun study is not an isolated case. Several other scientists have found that people who feel good live longer. But why would this be so? Some answers are emerging from the new field of positive psychology. This branch of psychological science surfaced about five years ago, as the brainchild of Martin E. P. Seligman, then president of the American Psychological Association (APA). Like many psychologists, Seligman had devoted much of his research

American Scientist, July–August 2003 v91 i4 p330(6)
"The Value of Positive Emotions: The Emerging Science of Positive Psychology Is Coming to Understand Why It's Good to Feel Good" by Barbara L. Fredrickson. © 2003 Sigma Xi, The Scientific Research Society

career to studying mental illness. He coined the phrase learned helplessness to describe how hopelessness and other negative thoughts can spiral down into clinical depression.

At the start of his term as APA president, Seligman took stock of the field of psychology, noting its significant advances in curing ills. In 1947, none of the major mental illnesses were treatable, whereas today 16 are treatable by psychotherapy, psychopharmacology or both. Although psychology had become proficient at rescuing people from various mental illnesses, it had virtually no scientifically sound tools for helping people to reach their higher ground, to thrive and flourish. Seligman aimed to correct this imbalance when he called for a "positive psychology." With the help of psychologist Mihaly Csikszentmihalyi—who originated the concept of "flow" to describe peak motivational experiences—Seligman culled the field for scientists whose work might be described as investigating "that which makes life worth living."

This is how many research psychologists, myself included, were drawn to positive psychology. My own background is in the study of emotions. For more than a dozen years, I've been studying the positive emotions—joy, contentment, gratitude and love—to shed light on their evolved adaptive significance. Among scientists who study emotions, this is a rare specialty. Far more emotion researchers have devoted their careers to studying negative emotions, such as anger, anxiety and sadness. The study of optimism and positive emotions was seen by some as a frivolous pursuit. But the positive psychology movement is changing that. Many psychologists have now begun to explore the largely uncharted terrain of human strengths and the sources of happiness.

The new discoveries generated by positive psychology hold the promise of improving individual and collective functioning, psychological well-being and physical health. But to harness the power of positive psychology, we need to understand how and why "goodness" matters. Although the discovery that people who think positively and feel good actually live longer is remarkable, it raises more questions than it answers. Exactly how do positive thinking and pleasant feelings help people live longer? Do pleasant thoughts and feelings help people live better as well? And why are positive emotions a universal part of human nature? My research traces the possible pathways for the life-enhancing effects of positive emotions and attempts to understand why human beings evolved to experience them.

WHY SO NEGATIVE?

There are probably a number of reasons why the positive emotions received little attention in the past. There is, of course, the natural tendency to study something that afflicts the well-being of humanity—and the expression and experience of negative emotions are responsible for much of what ails this world. But it may also be that the positive emotions are a little harder to study. They are comparatively few and relatively undifferentiated—joy, amusement and serenity are not easily distinguished from one another. Anger, fear and sadness, on the other hand, are distinctly different experiences.

This lack of differentiation is evident in how we think about the emotions. Consider that scientific taxonomies of basic emotions typically identify one positive emotion for every three or four negative emotions and that this imbalance is also reflected in the relative numbers of emotion words in the English language.

Various physical components of emotional expression similarly reveal a lack of differentiation for the positive emotions. The negative emotions have specific facial configurations that imbue them with universally recognized signal value. We can readily identify angry, sad or fearful faces. In contrast, facial expressions for positive emotions have no unique signal value: All share the Duchenne smile—in which the corners of the lips are raised and the muscles are contracted around the eyes, which raises the cheeks. A similar distinction is evident in the response of the autonomic nervous system to the expression of emotions. About 20 years ago, psychologists Paul Ekman and Wallace Friesen at the University of California, San Francisco, and Robert Levenson at Indiana University showed that anger, fear and sadness each elicit distinct responses in the autonomic nervous system. In contrast, the positive emotions appeared to have no distinguishable autonomic responses.

The study of positive emotions has also been hindered because scientists attempted to understand them with models that worked best for negative emotions. Central to many theories of emotion is that they are, by definition, associated with urges to act in particular ways. Anger creates the urge to attack, fear the urge to escape and disgust the urge to expectorate. Of course, no theorist argues that people invariably act out these urges; rather, people's ideas about possible courses of action narrow in on these specific urges. And these urges are not simply thoughts existing in the mind. They embody specific physiological changes that enable the actions called forth. In the case of fear, for example, a greater amount of blood flows to the large muscle groups to facilitate running.

The models that emphasize the role of these specific action tendencies typically cast the emotions as evolved adaptations. The negative emotions have an intuitively obvious adaptive value: In an instant, they narrow our thought-action repertoires to those that best promoted our ancestors' survival in life-threatening situations. In this view, negative emotions are efficient solutions to recurrent problems that our ancestors faced.

Positive emotions, on the other hand, aren't so easily explained. From this evolutionary perspective, joy, serenity and gratitude don't seem as useful as fear, anger or disgust. The bodily changes, urges to act and the facial expressions produced by positive emotions aren't as specific or as obviously relevant to survival as those sparked by negative emotions. If positive emotions didn't promote our ancestors' survival in life-threatening situations, then what good were they? Did they have any adaptive value at all? Perhaps they merely signaled the absence of threats.

THE BROADEN-AND-BUILD THEORY

We gain some insight into the adaptive role of positive emotions if we abandon the framework used to understand the negative emotions. Instead of solving problems of immediate survival, positive emotions solve problems concerning personal growth and development. Experiencing a positive emotion leads to states of mind and to modes of behavior that indirectly prepare an individual for later hard times. In my broaden-and-build theory, I propose that the positive emotions broaden an individual's momentary mindset, and by doing so help to build enduring personal resources. We can test these ideas by exploring the ways that positive emotions change how people think and how they behave.

My students and I conducted experiments in which we induced certain emotions in people by having them watch short, emotionally evocative film clips. We elicited joy by showing a herd of playful penguins waddling and sliding on the ice, we elicited serenity with clips of peaceful nature scenes, we elicited fear with films of people at precarious heights, and we elicited sadness with scenes of deaths and funerals. We also used a neutral "control" film of an old computer screen saver that elicited no emotion at all.

We then assessed the participant's ability to think broadly. Using global-local visual processing tasks, we measured whether they saw the "big picture" or focused on smaller details. The participant's task is to judge which of two comparison figures is more similar to a "standard" figure. Neither choice is right or wrong, but one comparison figure resembles the standard in global configuration, and the other in local, detailed elements. Using this and similar measures, we found that, compared to those in negative or neutral states, people who experience positive emotions (as assessed by self-report or electromyographic signals from the face) tend to choose the global configuration, suggesting a broadened pattern of thinking.

This tendency to promote a broader thought-action repertoire is linked to a variety of downstream effects of positive emotions on thinking. Two decades of experiments by Alice Isen of Cornell University and her colleagues have shown that people experiencing positive affect (feelings) think differently. One series of experiments tested creative thinking using such tests as Mednick's Remote Associates Test, which asks people to think of a word that relates to each of three other words. So, for example, given the words mower, atomic and foreign, the correct answer is power. Although this test was originally designed to assess individual differences in the presumably stable trait of creativity, Isen and colleagues showed that people experiencing positive affect perform better on this test than people in neutral states.

In other experiments, Isen and colleagues tested the clinical reasoning of practicing physicians. They made some of the physicians feel good by giving them a small bag of candy, then asked all of them to think aloud while they solved a case of a patient with liver disease. Content analyses revealed that physicians who felt good were faster to integrate case information and less likely to become anchored on initial thoughts or come to premature closure in their diagnosis. In yet another experiment, Isen and colleagues showed that negotiators induced to feel good were more likely to discover integrative solutions in a complex bargaining task. Overall, 20 years of experiments by Isen and her colleagues show that when people feel good, their thinking becomes more creative, integrative, flexible and open to information.

Even though positive emotions and the broadened mindsets they create are themselves short-lived, they can have deep and enduring effects. By momentarily broadening attention and thinking, positive emotions can lead to the discovery of novel ideas, actions and social bonds. For example, joy and playfulness build a variety of resources. Consider children at play in the schoolyard or adults enjoying a game of basketball in the gym. Although their immediate motivations may be simply hedonistic—to enjoy the moment—they are at the same time building physical, intellectual, psychological and social resources. The physical activity leads to long-term improvements in health, the game-playing strategies develop problem-solving skills, and the camaraderie strengthens social bonds that may provide crucial support at some time in the future. Similar links between playfulness and later gains in physical, social and intellectual resources are also evident in nonhuman animals, such as monkeys, rats and squirrels. In human beings, other positive states of mind and positive actions work along similar lines: Savoring an experience solidifies life priorities; altruistic acts strengthen social ties and build skills for expressing love and care. These outcomes often endure long after the initial positive emotion has vanished.

My students and I recently tested these ideas by surveying a group of people to examine their resilience and optimism. The people were originally interviewed in the early months of 2001, and then again in the days after the September 11th terrorist attacks. We asked them to identify the emotions they were feeling, what they had learned from the attacks and how optimistic they were about the future. We learned that after September 11 nearly everyone felt sad, angry and somewhat afraid. And more than 70 percent were depressed. Yet the people who were originally identified as being resilient in the early part of 2001 felt positive emotions strongly as well. They were also half as likely to be depressed. Our statistical analyses showed that their tendency to feel more positive emotions buffered the resilient people against depression.

Gratitude was the most common positive emotion people felt after the September 11th attacks. Feeling grateful was associated both with learning many good things from the crisis and with increased levels of optimism. Resilient people made statements such as, "I learned that most people in the world are inherently good." Put differently, feeling grateful broadened positive learning, which in turn built optimism, just as the broaden-and-build theory suggests.

My students and I have recently completed an experimental test of the building effect of positive emotions. Over the course of a month-long study of daily experiences, we induced one group of college students to feel more positive emotions by asking them to find the positive meaning and long-term benefit within their best, worst and seemingly ordinary experiences each day. At the end of the month, compared to others who did not make this daily effort to find positive meaning, those who did showed increases in psychological resilience.

So "feeling good" does far more than signal the absence of threats. It can transform people for the better, making them more optimistic, resilient and socially connected. Indeed, this insight might solve the evolutionary mystery of positive emotions: Simply by experiencing positive emotions, our ancestors would have naturally accrued more personal resources. And when later faced with threats to life or limb, these greater resources translated into greater odds of survival and greater odds of living long enough to reproduce.

THE UNDOING HYPOTHESIS

We might also ask whether there are other immediate benefits to experiencing positive emotions, aside from the tautology that they make us "feel good." One effect relates to how people cope with their negative emotions. If negative emotions narrow people's mindsets and positive emotions broaden them, then perhaps positive emotions undo the lingering effects of negative emotions.

Such effects may extend to the physiological realm. The negative emotions have distinct physiological responses associated with them—autonomic activity (as mentioned earlier), including cardiovascular activity, which represents the body's preparation for specific action. A number of studies suggest that the cardiovascular activity associated with stress and negative emotions, especially if prolonged and recurrent, can promote or exacerbate heart disease. Experiments on nonhuman primates reveal that recurrent emotion-related cardiovascular activity also appears to injure the inner walls of arteries and initiate atherosclerosis. Because the positive emotions broaden people's thought-and-action repertoires, they may also loosen the hold that negative emotions gain on both mind and body, dismantle preparation for specific action and undo the physiological effects of negative emotions.

My colleagues and I tested this undoing hypothesis in a series of experiments. We began by inducing a negative emotion: We told participants that they had one minute to prepare a speech that would be videotaped and evaluated by their peers. The speech task induced the subjective feeling of anxiety as well as increases in heart rate, peripheral vasoconstriction and blood pressure. We then randomly assigned the participants to view one of four films: two films evoked mild positive emotions (amusement and contentment), a third served as a neutral control condition and a fourth elicited sadness.

We then measured the time elapsed from the beginning of the randomly assigned film until the cardiovascular reactions induced by the speech task returned to each participant's baseline levels. The results were consistent:

Those individuals who watched the two positive-emotion films recovered to their baseline cardiovascular activity sooner than those who watched the neutral film. Those who watched the sad film showed the most delayed recovery. Positive emotions had a clear and consistent effect of undoing the cardiovascular repercussions of negative emotions.

At this point the cognitive and physiological mechanisms of the undoing effect are unknown. It may be that broadening one's cognitive perspective by feeling positive emotions mediates the physiological undoing. Such ideas need further exploration.

ENDING ON A POSITIVE NOTE

So how do the positive emotions promote longevity? Why did the happy nuns live so long? It seems that positive emotions do more than simply feel good in the present. The undoing effect suggests that positive emotions can reduce the physiological "damage" on the cardiovascular system sustained by feeling negative emotions. But some other research suggests that there's more to it than that. It appears that experiencing positive emotions increases the likelihood that one will feel good in the future.

My colleague Thomas Joiner and I sought to test whether positive affect and broadened thinking mutually enhance each other—so that experiencing one produces the other, which in turn encourages more of the first one, and so on in a mutually reinforcing ascent to greater well-being. We measured positive affect and broadened thinking strategies in 138 college students on two separate occasions, five weeks apart (times T1 and T2), with standard psychological tests. When we compared the students' responses on both occasions we found some very interesting results: Positive affect at T1 predicted increases in both positive affect and broadened thinking at T2; and broadened thinking at TI predicted increases in both positive affect and broadened thinking at T2. Further statistical analyses revealed that there was indeed a mutually reinforcing effect between positive affect and broadened thinking. These results suggest that people who regularly feel positive emotions are in some respects lifted on an "upward spiral" of continued growth and thriving.

But positive emotions don't just transform individuals. I've argued that they may also transform groups of people, within communities and organizations. Community transformation becomes possible because each person's positive emotion can resound through others. Take helpful, compassionate acts as an example. Isen demonstrated that people who experience positive emotions become more helpful to others. Yet being helpful not only springs from positive emotions, it also produces positive emotions. People who give help, for instance, can feel proud of their good deeds and so experience continued good feelings. Plus, people who receive help can feel grateful, and those who merely witness good deeds can feel elevated. Each of these positive emotions—pride, gratitude and elevation—can in turn broaden people's mindsets and inspire further compassionate acts. So, by creating chains of events that carry positive meaning for others, positive emotions can trigger upward spirals that transform communities into more cohesive, moral and harmonious social organizations.

All of this suggests that we need to develop methods to experience more positive emotions more often. Although the use of humor, laughter and other direct attempts to stimulate positive emotions are occasionally suitable, they often seem poor choices, especially in trying times. Based on our recent experiment with college students, my advice would be to cultivate positive emotions indirectly by finding positive meaning within current circumstances. Positive meaning can be obtained by finding benefits within adversity, by infusing ordinary events with meaning and by effective problem solving. You can find benefits in a grim world, for instance, by focusing on the newfound strengths and resolve within yourself and others. You can infuse ordinary events with meaning by expressing appreciation, love and gratitude, even for simple things. And you can find positive meaning through problem solving by supporting compassionate acts toward people in need. So although the active ingredient within growth and resilience may be positive emotions, the leverage point for accessing these benefits is finding positive meaning.

So, what good is it to think about the good in the world? The mind can be a powerful ally. As John Milton told us, "The mind is its own place, and in itself can make a heaven of hell, a hell of heaven." The new science of positive psychology is beginning to unravel how such transformations can take place. Think about the good in the world, or otherwise find positive meaning, and you seed your own positive emotions. A focus on goodness cannot only change your life and your community, but perhaps also the world, and in time create a heaven on earth.

BIBLIOGRAPHY

Aspinwall, L. G., and U. M. Staudinger. 2003. *A Psychology of Human Strengths: Fundamental Questions and Future Directions for a Positive Psychology*. Washington, D.C.: American Psychological Association.

Danner, D. D., D. A. Snowdon and W. V. Friesen. 2001. Positive emotions in early life and longevity: Findings from the nun study. *Journal of Personality and Social Psychology* 80:804–813.

Fredrickson, B. L. 1998. What good are positive emotions? *Review of General Psychology* 2:300–319.

Fredrickson, B. L. 2000. Cultivating positive emotions to optimize health and well-being. *Prevention and Treatment* 3. http://journals.apa.org/prevention/volume3//toc-mar07–00.html

Fredrickson, B. L. 2001. The role of positive emotions in positive psychology: The broaden-and-build theory of positive emotions. *American Psychologist* 56:218–226.

Fredrickson, B. L., and T. Joiner. 2002. Positive emotions trigger upward spirals toward emotional well-being. *Psychological Science* 13:172–175.

Fredrickson, B. L., and R. W. Levenson. 1998. Positive emotions speed recovery from the cardiovascular sequelae of negative emotions. *Cognition and Emotion* 12:291–220.

Fredrickson, B. L., M. M. Tugade, C. E. Waugh and G. Larkin. 2003. What good are positive emotions in crises?: A prospective study of resilience and emotions following the terrorist attacks on the United States on September 11th, 2001. *Journal of Personality and Social Psychology* 84:365–376.

Isen, A. M. 1987. Positive affect, cognitive processes and social behavior. *Advances in Experimental Social Psychology* 20:203–253.

DISCUSSION QUESTIONS

1. At the beginning of the article the author describes a study conducted on Catholic nuns. What did this early study reveal about positive emotions and life expectancy?

2. What are some of the goals and objectives of positive psychology?

3. What does the broaden-and-build theory propose with respect to positive emotions?

4. What were the findings of the September 11th study the author discusses?

5. How does the author think positive emotions promote longevity?

2

The Impact of a Health Campaign on Hand Hygiene and Upper Respiratory Illness Among College Students Living in Residence Halls

Cindy White, Robin Kolble, Rebecca Carlson, and Natasha Lipson

Abstract: Hand hygiene is a key element in preventing the transmission of cold and flu viruses. The authors conducted an experimental-control design study in 4 campus residence halls to determine whether a message campaign about hand hygiene and the availability of gel hand sanitizer could decrease cold and flu illness and school and work absenteeism. Their findings indicate that students who were exposed to the message campaign and provided with gel hand sanitizer increased their knowledge about the potential health benefits of hand washing and sanitizer use; they reported higher rates

Journal of American College Health, Jan–Feb 2005 v53 i4 p175(7).
"The Impact of a Health Campaign on Hand Hygiene and Upper Respiratory Illness Among College Students Living in Residence Halls" by Cindy White, Robin Kolble, Rebecca Carlson, and Natasha Lipson. © 2005 Heldref Publications

of hand washing and using sanitizer than did the control group. These students also experienced fewer cold and flu illnesses during the study than those in the control group and missed fewer class or work engagements because of colds or flu. Conducting a health promotion campaign in residence halls may therefore help prevent colds and flu and decrease absenteeism on university campuses.

INTRODUCTION

Hand hygiene is a key element in preventing the transmission of cold and flu viruses. The authors conducted an experimental-control design study in 4 campus residence halls to determine whether a message campaign about hand hygiene and the availability of gel hand sanitizer could decrease cold and flu illness and school and work absenteeism. Their findings indicate that students who were exposed to the message campaign and provided with gel hand sanitizer increased their knowledge about the potential health benefits of hand washing and sanitizer use; they reported higher rates of hand washing and using sanitizer than did the control group. These students also experienced fewer cold and flu illnesses during the study than those in the control group and missed fewer class or work engagements because of colds or flu. Conducting a health promotion campaign in residence halls may therefore help prevent colds and flu and decrease absenteeism on university campuses.

Upper respiratory infections (URIs) are a common experience among college students. Reducing URIs on college campuses is important for 3 reasons. First, young adults face a greater likelihood of experiencing illness from colds and flu. Two studies conducted among medical students and workers in an insurance company revealed a significantly higher frequency of URIs among young adults than that reported by researchers who looked at a more general population. (1) The likelihood of experiencing a URI may be even greater for college students, who live in group environments such as residence halls. (2) Second, college health centers often must devote many resources to assisting students with URIs. At the university where this study was conducted, the Health Center staff saw 3,121 students for URI symptoms during the 2001 fall semester. A number of those students had viral infections that did not require medical intervention and would go away without treatment. Third, there is evidence that students' illnesses have a negative influence on their academic performance. According to the American College Health Association's (ACHA) spring 2002 National College Health Assessment (NCHA), 22% of students reported that "cold/flu/sore throat" had a negative impact on their academic performance, and 8% reported "sinus infections" as an impediment to their academic performance. (3) Thus, reducing the occurrence of URIs may benefit students and assist health promotion programs in improving students' health and academic success.

Before we conducted this study, the Community Health Education Department and the Medical Clinic at our health center collaborated to reduce the incidence of URIs among students. Staff members from the Student Wellness Program distributed educational materials explaining how to prevent and treat symptoms of URIs, distinguish the common cold from other, more serious upper respiratory infections, and gain access to care. They also provided "cold care kits" to students on campus to encourage self-care. In addition, the medical clinic established a walk-in cold clinic and designed protocols for directing patients to the appropriate clinician for care. But one important goal of the health center was to help students learn to prevent URI illness.

The Centers for Disease Control and Prevention (CDC) and the Association for Professionals in Infection Control and Epidemiology maintain that simple hand washing is the single most important and effective method of preventing disease transmission. (4,5) Hand washing is defined as vigorous and brief rubbing together of all surfaces of soap-lathered hands, followed by rinsing under a stream of water. (6) Alcohol-based hand sanitizers provide a convenient adjunct to hand washing. These products do not remove soil or organic material, but do kill microorganisms through disinfectant action. (6) Previous research has demonstrated that improving hand hygiene can decrease URIs. For example, Hammond and associates (7) reported that a hand-hygiene regimen in elementary schools that incorporated Purell hand sanitizer was successful in decreasing absenteeism resulting from illness. In a study of preschool children, Carabin and associates (8) found that increasing the frequency of individuals' washing their hands decreased the incidence of both URI and gastrointestinal illness. Naval recruits in basic training who participated in a program that mandated hand washing at least 5 times daily were found to have a significantly reduced incidence of URI. (9) In this study, we sought to discover whether a campaign to increase hand hygiene practices, coupled with the introduction of an alcohol-based antibacterial gel, reinforced by messages to continue washing and sanitizing, would decrease the incidence of URI in a residence hall population on the campus of a major western university. We anticipated that an increase in hand-hygiene would reduce the number of reported URIs.

METHOD

Study Design

This study involved an experimental-control group design. We recruited students from 4 on-campus residence halls as participants. We selected the 4 residences because the hall directors were willing to assist with the study and because the residence students were typical of students in on-campus residence halls. However, we did make an attempt to match halls on 1 key factor—academic emphasis. Two of the residence halls included academic programs as part of their learning environment, so we assigned 1 of these halls to the experimental group and 1 to the control group. The other 2 halls had no special emphasis: we assigned 1 to the experimental group and 1 to the control group.

Participants in the experimental halls were exposed to a health campaign designed to increase awareness of the importance of hand washing and hand cleanliness in avoiding colds and the flu. Residents (both study participants and nonparticipants) in the experimental hall also received free Purell hand sanitizer in their rooms and in travel packs; gel hand sanitizer was also available in the dormitory bathrooms and just inside the hall dining room. Students in the control residence were told that they were participating in at study to examine wellness behaviors and their links to illness. This was a reasonable explanation of the investigation because the study examined a number of health behaviors.

All participants completed pre- and poststudy surveys regarding knowledge, attitudes, and behaviors related to various health practices. They also completed weekly surveys that provided reports of their experience of cold or flu symptoms, use of tobacco and exercise habits, hand washing, and use of gel sanitizers. We conducted the study in September, October, and November and collected weekly reports from students for each of 8 weeks.

Participants

Participants were students who lived in selected campus residence halls, each of which housed 300 to 400 students. Our goal was to recruit 100 students in each hall for a total of approximately 400 participants; we chose this number because a sample of approximately 400 provided a good estimation of student behavior in each hall and was large enough to detect moderate effects in comparing the experimental and control groups. (10) Initially, 430 students enrolled in the study. However, not all would-be participants completed each portion of the study. To be included in the data analyses, a participant had to complete the prestudy measures and 3 weekly reports of illness behavior; 391 participants met these criteria for inclusion in analyses (188 participants in experimental condition: 203 in control condition).

Measures

We used 3 sets of surveys designed to discover particular aspects of this study: (1) pre- and posttest surveys, (2) weekly surveys, and (3) message-recall surveys. Pre- and postsurveys examined participants' knowledge, attitudes, and perceived behaviors related to a healthy lifestyle, the impact of hand hygiene on wellness, and basic demographic information. Weekly surveys inquired about URI symptoms and daily hand hygiene, smoking, and exercise regimens. Message surveys were distributed to the experimental group midway through the research project and as part of the poststudy survey to explore information on attitudes toward and retention of the hand-health messages posted in the experimental residence halls.

It is important to note that the study provided an opportunity to gather 2 types of behavioral data. In the pre- and postsurveys, we gathered information about perceived behaviors: that is, we asked the participants how often they thought they typically engaged in the behavior. For instance, we asked if they washed their hands before eating a meal all the time, most of the time, some of the time, rarely, or never. In the weekly surveys, we were able to gather more specific information about behavior for the specific day or week. Thus, we asked participants how many times, since getting up in the morning, they had washed their hands on that particular day. Although both of these reports relied on participants' recall of their own behavior, the perceived behavior measures told us what participants believed they did, and the measure of daily behavior provided a more precise report of specific behavior for a single day.

Pre/Poststudy Assessment of Knowledge, Attitudes, and Behavior

The pre- and poststudy surveys gathered information about knowledge, attitudes, and behaviors regarding (1) hand hygiene, (2) exercise, (3) nutrition, (4) sleep behavior, (5) stress, and (6) exercise. We interspersed items related to each of these behaviors to ensure that the control group participants viewed the study as assessing general wellness. In addition, participants completed measures of social support related to health behaviors and general social support from resident hall members, friends, and family, as well as a measure of adjustment to college. We present a brief summary of each measure used in our analysis; readers can get further information on other measures from us. We assessed knowledge about hand hygiene with 6 objective items (true, false, and don't know were the options). These items asked about the effectiveness of hand washing in removing germs that could cause illness (e.g., washing your hands with soap and water can remove up to 99% of the germs on your hands), the spread of illness (e.g., if you sit near someone with a cold or flu, you are likely to catch it), and the use of gel sanitizers (e.g., gel sanitizers kill 99% of germs). The responses provided an assessment of participants' understanding of URI transmission and the role of hand hygiene in preventing the spread of URI.

We used a Likert-type scale to assess attitudes toward hand hygiene with 3 items: (1) it is easy to wash my, hands regularly; (2) washing helps me stay well; and (3) washing is an important health behavior. This scale achieved adequate reliability (Cronbach's $\alpha = .70$). We assessed attitudes toward gel sanitizer with 4 items that were reliable (Cronbach's $\alpha = .70$). Three of the items were the same as the washing items but referred to gel hand sanitizers. The fourth item asked whether participants viewed gel sanitizers as feeling sticky; we included this item because a pilot study we conducted indicated that the physical sensation of sanitizers influenced students' willingness to use the product.

In addition, we assessed perceived behavior for hand hygiene, nutrition (eating habits), exercise, and smoking. Behavioral questions asked participants to report their perceived frequency of engaging in a behavior (all the time, most of the time, sometimes, rarely, and never). To assess hand-washing behavior, we used 8 items. The scale achieved an overall reliability of .79 (Cronbach's α). The items asked about washing before and after meals, before snacking or preparing food, after sneezing or coughing, after petting an animal, and after shaking hands.

Weekly Surveys

After initial enrollment, participants completed the survey once a week for 8 weeks; they could complete the survey on paper or on the Internet link of the campus health center Web site. The weekly survey inquired about the presence and duration of 8 URI symptoms: sore throat, stuffy or runny nose, ear pain, painful or swollen neck, chest cough, chest congestion, sinus pressure, pain, and fever. For each symptom, participants indicated whether they had experienced the symptom in the previous week, and if so, how long the symptom had lasted. The survey also asked about frequency and timing of hand washing and sanitizer use. Specifically, participants were asked to recall the number of times they had washed their hands or used a gel sanitizer since waking. We also asked whether participants had missed class, work, or recreational activities because of URI symptoms, and if so, for how many days. Additional questions asked about the days of the week that participants had smoked cigarettes and exercised in the previous week.

Message Effectiveness

We administered message-recall surveys to the experimental group at the midpoint and at the end of the study. These questionnaires asked if and where students had seen messages regarding hand hygiene, the nature of the most memorable message, the impact of the messages, and whether they had discussed hand hygiene with anyone in their residence hall.

Procedure

We designed all surveys, and the Institutional Review Board at the university reviewed and approved the study. We recruited participants through e-mails and fliers distributed to residents of the selected residence halls. Both the fliers and e-mails explained the nature of the study and listed the incentives for participation. Enrollment was entirely voluntary, and students could discontinue participation at any time.

Enrollment and Incentives

During the enrollment session, students completed consent forms describing the nature of the study and were assigned a confidential number that they were to use on every response; it allowed them to access the Web-based survey each week. Participants also completed the pretest on knowledge, attitude, and behavior. We gave them $5 for each survey they completed, $5 for enrolling, and $20 extra if they completed all 8 surveys, summing to a maximum of $65 for perfect reporting. We distributed monetary incentives at the midpoint and at the end of the study. Participants also received weekly e-mail reminders about the study and nonmonetary incentives (such as pizza coupons) that were designed to encourage them to continue participating.

Message Design

We used Rogers' innovation–diffusion theory (11) as a guide in developing the health messages. This theory identifies the stages an individual passes through when adopting a new behavior: (1) knowing about the behavior, (2) forming an attitude toward the behavior, (3) making a decision to adopt or reject the behavior, (4) implementing the new idea, and (5) confirming the decision. We focused first on gaining student attention and providing information about hand hygiene that would increase their knowledge about potential benefits of adopting this behavior. To initiate the message campaign, we displayed bulletin boards entitled "Top 10 gross things students have on their hands" in the hall corridors and outside dining halls; this message sought to gain student attention and stimulate discussion by playing on the top-10 format and by mentioning behavior with which students might identify but would find mildly offensive (e.g., nose picking).

We also placed flier messages in the bathroom stalls of the experimental group and changed the messages weekly. The messages progressed from attention getting to knowledge, benefits, and persuasion. The first 4 weekly messages in the restrooms focused on introducing the benefits of hand washing, using hand sanitizers, and increasing participants' awareness of the positive effects of and hygiene and use of hand-sanitizer gel. Examples included a message that told students that most common infections are transmitted to others by touching contaminated surfaces. Messages during the second of the 4 weeks concentrated oil persuading participants to continue sanitizer use and hand washing by presenting some positive outcomes of clean hands (e.g., staying healthy leads to more time to socialize and to get better grades). Before the study began, student focus groups had examined and discussed the weekly messages to determine which ones they considered most effective.

Hand Washing and Sanitizer Use Rates

We calculated the score used to assess hand washing or gel hand sanitizer use on the basis of the average number of times since waking that particular day that participants reported washing or using sanitizer. We divided it by the number of hours participants had been awake that day to create a ratio of washings or sanitizer use per hour. For example, a participant who had been awake for 8 hours and had washed 3 times would receive a wash score of .375. In some cases, students completed the survey shortly after waking, which produced a hand-health ratio of 1.0 or greater. When this happened, we dropped the student's score for that week from our analyses. Although recall of specific behavior is always tricky, we expected that students would be able to think back through their days and provide reasonable estimates of hand washing and sanitizer use. Because we gathered data from each participant over 8 weeks, we were able to generate an average washing score and an average sanitizer score that we believed might provide a more stable assessment of behavior.

RESULTS

The university requires that first-year students live in the residence halls, so the majority of our population consisted of college freshmen (85.6%). More female (61.9%) than male students (38.1%) enrolled in the study. An overwhelming majority of our population was White (88%), and smaller numbers identified themselves as African American (1.7%), Hispanic or Latino (4.2%), Asian or Pacific Islander (2.8%), or Native or Alaskan American (.3%); 3% of participants did not report race. We found no significant demographic differences between participants in the experimental and control groups, and no difference between these groups in terms of reported experience of seasonal allergies or smoking behavior. Living arrangements in each hall were similar, although the average number of roommates for participants in the experimental group was 1, whereas the average number of roommates for participants in the control group was .87. Although this difference was statistically significant, we did not believe that it reflected an important difference in actual living arrangements for most participants.

Pre/Poststudy Reports of Knowledge, Attitudes, and Perceived Behavior

Data in Table 1 present our findings regarding changes in knowledge, attitudes, and perceived behavior. We used a repeated measures analysis of variance (ANOVA) to assess changes in these factors. As expected, knowledge about hand hygiene increased in the experimental group but not in the control group, $F(1, 334) = 11.25$, $p < .001$. Attitudes toward hand washing increased over time in both the experimental and control groups, $F(1, 342) = 19.76$, $p < .001$. No main effect for Condition or Time x Condition interaction emerged. Attitudes toward the health benefit of gel sanitizers revealed only a main effect for condition. $F(1, 342) = 34.46$, $p < .001$, with participants in the experimental group expressing more positive attitudes toward gel sanitizers than participants in the control group.

TABLE 1   Pre- and Poststudy Attitudes, Knowledge, and Perceived Behavior in a Health Campaign on Hand Hygiene and Upper Respiratory Illness

	Group							
	Experimental				Control			
	Prestudy		Poststudy		Prestudy		Poststudy	
Variable	M	SD	M	SD	M	SD	M	SD
Knowledge	4.56	1.26	5.14	.98	4.62	1.10	4.70	1.34
Hand-washing attitude	3.82	.06	4.03	.05	3.96	.05	4.06	.05
Sanitizer attitude	3.47	.06	3.52	.06	3.10	.06	3.07	.06
Perceived behavior	2.87	.04	2.80	.05	2.81	.05	2.83	.05

The measure of participants' perceived hand–hygiene behavior involved questions about the perceived frequency with which participants washed their hands before eating a meal (all of the time, most of the time, sometimes, rarely and never). We think of this scale as reflecting perceived hand–health behavior because it provides a general assessment of the extent to which participants believe they engage in the behavior. A main effect for time emerged, $F(1, 325) = 21.14$, $p < .0001$, $\beta^2 = .06$, with perceived hand-washing behavior increasing from the prestudy assessment to the poststudy assessment in both conditions (lower scores reflect more frequent behavior).

Weekly Data Regarding Washing Behavior, Sanitizer Use, and Illness

Our analyses of the data culled from the weekly reports revealed that the experimental group had significantly better hand hygiene than did the control group (see Table 2). This reflected a difference in both hand-washing behavior, $t(330) = 2.06$, $p < .02$, and hand-sanitizer use between experimental and control halls, $t(367) = 12.92$, $p < .0001$. We also examined whether women and men differed in their hand-hygiene practices. Analyses of variance revealed

TABLE 2   Hand Washing and Sanitizer Use Rates in a Study of Upper Respiratory Illness Among College Students

| | Rates/hour | |
Group	Hand Washing	Sanitizer Use
Experimental	.48	.26
Control	.43	.03

that women washed their hands more frequently than men did (.49 vs .40), $F(1,295) = 11.60$, $p < .001$, but did not differ significantly in their use of gel hand sanitizer.

The weekly data also revealed differences in illness rates between the experimental and control groups. On the basis of self-reported symptoms from the weekly reports, we identified students as experiencing an upper respiratory infection when they reported having 2 or more URI symptoms that lasted at least 2 to 3 days. (9) The experimental group reported 26% fewer illnesses than the control group; the illness rate for the experimental group was 20.2%, whereas it was 27.5% for the control group across the study, $\chi^2 = 19.97$, $p < .0001$.

Absenteeism

We measured absenteeism by asking participants to report in their weekly surveys whether they had missed school, work, or recreational activities as a result of upper respiratory symptoms. To complete this analysis, we combined reports of school and work and compared the experimental and control groups. Significantly more participants in the control group reported missing at least 1 day of school or work because of illness (9.5%), compared with the product-use group (5.7%), $\chi^2 = 13.39$, $p < .0001$; this reflects 40% fewer absences in the experimental group compared with the control group.

Message Campaign

The effectiveness of the message campaign was partially reflected in participants' improved knowledge about hand hygiene that we gathered in pre- and postsurveys at the midpoint and end of the study. We also assessed whether students had encountered the hand-hygiene messages, which aspects of the campaign they found, and their perceptions of the campaign. The majority of students in the experimental group (76%) indicated that they had encountered a message in their residence hall about hand washing. Reports of where students had encountered the messages indicated that the messages in the bathrooms were most visible (96% of students had encountered them). The messages on bulletin boards on residence hall floors and in common areas were seen by many students (56% and 54%, respectively), but clearly not as often as the messages in the bathrooms.

Analyses of the perceptions of the message indicated that students saw the messages as containing accurate, interesting, and useful information. The messages were also generally seen as good reminders and as relatively encouraging (see Table 3). In addition, we asked whether the messages led students to talk about hand hygiene with others in their residence halls because we anticipated that generating conversations among students would heighten awareness and reinforce behavior. Reports indicated that 32% of the respondents had talked about hand washing with someone in their residence hall during the last month (the duration of the study up to that point).

TABLE 3   Perceptions of a Hand-Hygiene Message Campaign

Characteristic of message	M
Accurate/correct information	1.80
Interesting information	1.73
Useful information	2.00
Good reminders	2.04
Encouraging	2.17

NOTE: Ratings were on a 4-point scale with lower numbers indicative of the most positive reaction to the campaign.

COMMENT

We examined whether URIs among college students living in residence halls could be reduced through a message campaign that promoted hand hygiene and made gel hand sanitizer available to students. In comparing the experimental and control groups, we found that students in the experimental condition who received the message campaign and gel sanitizer washed their hands and used gel sanitizer more often than those in the control group. They also experienced fewer URIs and missed fewer classes and work as a result of URIs.

Participants in the experimental group increased their knowledge about the nature of hand hygiene and the spread of URI from the pre- to poststudy assessments. Positive attitudes toward hand washing and sanitizer use increased during the study for participant in both the control and experimental groups. Although we expected that positive attitudes would increase more in the experimental than in the control group, we believe this change occurred for 2 reasons: (1) attitudes were relatively positive to begin with (approaching 4 on a 5-point scale), so there may have been a ceiling effect that allowed little room for attitude change: (2) the questions in the prestudy survey and the weekly survey, although mixed with many other health behavior items, could have led students to think more positively about hand hygiene. We believe this finding is interesting because it suggests that simply making students aware of a behavior could have a positive impact on their attitudes toward it.

The messages we used in this study first focused on increasing knowledge about hand hygiene and URI transmission, then tried to reinforce the benefits of avoiding URIs. Participants reported that they viewed the messages as accurate and relevant, and they said that they had noticed the messages throughout the halls. Interpreted from the perspective of a diffusion-of-innovations model, (11) these data indicated that the messages were likely to have an impact because they heightened awareness of hand hygiene and created a situation that resulted in at least some students discussing the issue.

Recent data from the American College Health Association (ACHA) study (3) suggest that illness has a negative impact on students' academic performance and that URIs are often the culprit. This negative effect of illness on academic success may be particularly strong for first-year students who live in residence halls because of the challenges of their transition to college. Programs that help students avoid illness can play an important role in supporting the university's mission. Our findings suggest that the health of students in residence halls can be improved through a hand-hygiene program designed to increase student knowledge about the benefits of hand washing and sanitizer use.

Limitations

Although this study indicates this program's positive effect on illness rates and hand-hygiene knowledge, several limitations should be noted. First, the study demonstrates the combined impact of a campaign that focuses on the benefits of hand hygiene and the availability of gel sanitizer. Thus, it is not possible to determine whether the message campaign or sanitizer alone would influence illness. We chose to implement a message campaign along with sanitizer for 2 reasons. First, we wanted to encourage both hand washing and sanitizer use. In light of a recent CDC discussion, we believe that hand sanitizers are a good supplement for hand hygiene, but they cannot replace hand washing. We wanted to ensure that students understood the importance of both washing and using a sanitizer. Second, we did not expect that simply making sanitizer available to students would change their behaviors. Focus groups we had conducted with students, as well as a previous pilot study, suggested that students needed to be encouraged to engage in good hand hygiene.

Another limitation stems from the use of self-report data. We did not verify illness by medical examination, so it is possible that some students experienced symptoms and were classified as having an illness when they were not ill. Self-reports have been used in other studies of this type, primarily because they are an expedient way to gather data from larger samples. However, additional research that uses health-center visits or medical records could be used to examine the influence of hand hygiene on URI. Because we had no baseline rates of illness in each residence hall, we could not determine whether some differences in illness may have resulted from the overall illness rate in each hall, but we have no reason to believe that these halls would vary in their baseline illness rates.

Finally, the likelihood of contracting a URI is influenced by a number of health behaviors. Although careful hand hygiene can help students avoid URIs, other health behaviors probably determine whether an individual contracts a URI. At this point, we have examined smoking and allergy rates because they have a direct link to upper respiratory health. We found no difference in smoking or allergy rates between the experimental and control groups. As we anticipated, smoking slightly increased the occurrence of URI in both groups. We are further examining the data to determine how other behaviors, such as exercise and diet, affect students' health.

Decreases in URIs and absenteeism are significant because healthy students contribute to meeting the mission of the university. URIs among the college population have a negative effect on students' ability to attend classes, concentrate on their studies and work, and participate in social activities. Thus, URIs can affect students' academic achievement and retention. The findings in this study demonstrate that health campaigns that promote hand hygiene can reduce student illness and absenteeism and contribute to the health of the student community; they also suggest that students have relatively positive attitudes toward good hand hygiene and indicate that campaigns designed to influence students' behavior need not be complex. Such campaigns need to inform students about the benefits of good hand hygiene and encourage the practice. We believe the results of this study provide strong arguments for implementing similar hand-hygiene campaigns at other universities to foster students' health and success.

REFERENCES

1. Barker J, Stevens D, Bloomfield SF. Spread and prevention of some common viral infections in community facilities and domestic homes. *J Appl Microbiol.* 2001;91:7–21.

2. Moe CL, Christmas WA, Echols LJ, Miller SE. Outbreaks of acute gastroenteritis associated with Norwalk-like viruses in campus settings. *J Am Coil Health.* 2001:50:57–66.

3. American College Health Association. The NCHA Web Summary page. Available at: http://www.acha.org/projects_ programs/ncha_sampledata_public.cfm. Accessed June 26, 2003.

4. Boyce JM, Pittet D. Guideline for hand hygiene in healthcare settings. *MMWR.* 2002;51 (RR 16):1–44.

5. Larson EL. APIC guidelines for hand washing and hand antisepsis in healthcare settings. *Am J Infect Control.* 1995:23:251–269.

6. Widmer AF. Replace hand washing with use of a waterless alcohol band rub? *Clin Infect Dis.* 2000;31:36–43.

7. Hammond B, Ali Y, Fendler E, Dolan M, Donovan S. Effect of hand sanitizer use on elementary school absenteeism. *Am J Infect Control.* 2000;28(5):340–346.

8. Carabin H, Gyorkos TW, Soto JC, Joseph L, Payment P, Collet J-R Effectiveness of a training program in reducing infections in toddlers attending day care centers. *Epidemiology.* 1999:10:219–227.

9. Ryan MAK, Christian RS, Wohlrabe J. Hand washing and respiratory illness among young adults in military training. *Am J Prev Med.* 2001:21(2):79–83.

10. Rosenthal R, Rosnow RL. *Essentials of Behavioral Research: Methods and Data Analysis.* 2nd ed. New York: McGraw-Hill; 1991.

11. Rogers E. *Diffusion of Innovations.* 4th ed. New York: Johns Hopkins Press; 1995.

DISCUSSION QUESTIONS

1. What is the purpose of this study?
2. What is the independent variable in this study?
3. What are the dependent variables in this study? (Hint: There may be more than one)
4. What did the researchers find (i.e., what was the affect of the independent variable on the dependent variables?)
5. What are the limitations of this study?

3

Extending the Theory of Planned Behavior in the Exercise Domain: A Comparison of Social Support and Subjective Norm

Ryan E. Rhodes, Lee W. Jones, and Kerry S. Courneya

Ajzen's (1991) theory of planned behavior (TPB) has emerged as one of the dominant social cognitive frameworks for understanding exercise motivation and behavior. The TPB provides a parsimonious explanation of informational and motivational influences on behavior and can be considered a deliberative processing model. The hypothesized proximal determinant of volitional behavior is one's intention to engage in that behavior. Intentions reflect a conscious plan or decision to enact the behavior. The TPB tries also to predict incompletely volitional behaviors by incorporating perceptions of control over performance of the behavior as an additional predictor

Research Quarterly for Exercise and Sport, June 2002 v73 i2 p193(7).
"Extending the Theory of Planned Behavior in the Exercise Domain: A Comparison of Social Support and Subjective Norm" by Ryan E. Rhodes, Lee W. Jones, and Kerry S. Courneya. © 2002 American Alliance for Health, Physical Education, Recreation and Dance (AAHPERD)

(Ajzen, 1991). Perceived behavioral control (PBC) is the individual's perception of the extent to which performance of the behavior is easy or difficult (Ajzen, 1991). Further, PBC is also hypothesized to influence behavior indirectly through intentions, along with attitudes and subjective norms. Attitudes are the individual's overall evaluations of performing the behavior. Subjective norms consist of a person's beliefs about whether significant others think he or she should engage in the behavior and are assumed to assess the social pressures on the individual to perform or not to perform a particular behavior.

Quantitative reviews have consistently supported the utility of the TPB in the exercise domain (Godin & Kok, 1996; Hausenblaus, Carron, & Mack, 1997). However, the construct of subjective norm has not performed well in explaining exercise intentions across studies when controlling for attitude and PBC, typically being either nonsignificant or of small significant magnitude. Given the poor performance of subjective norm in exercise research, some researchers have suggested that it may not be the most theoretically relevant social influence construct in the exercise domain (Courneya & McAuley, 1995a, 1995b; Courneya, Plotnikoff, Hotz, & Birkett, 2000). Courneya and colleagues (Courneya & McAuley, 1995a, 1995b; Courneya et al., 2000) have argued that social support may provide for a greater understanding of exercise motivation and behavior.

The conceptual distinction between these two social influence constructs is that subjective norm refers to the perceived pressure to perform a behavior that comes from observing what important others say or do, whereas social support implies the perception of assistance in performing the behavior (Courneya et al., 2000). The theoretical argument of Courneya et al. (2000) for why social support should be superior to subjective norm in the exercise domain is due to exercise behavior not being under complete volitional control (i.e., not capable of being done at will, or free of practical constraints). That is, subjective norm may be the most relevant social influence construct for behaviors that are under complete volitional control, because for such behaviors a person only needs to know whether important others approve of the behavior. By definition, they do not need any help. For behaviors that are incompletely volitional, however (e.g., exercise), it is likely that assistance from others for performing the behavior (i.e., social support) would be helpful beyond knowing they approve of the behavior. Any relationship between these concepts is hypothesized to occur from common exogenous concepts, similar to the tenets of relationships between attitude, subjective norm, and PBC in the TPB proper (Ajzen, 1991).

Only two studies have directly compared the relative utility of subjective norm and social support in the exercise domain (Courneya & McAuley, 1995a; Courneya et al., 2000), and, unfortunately, both have significant limitations. Courneya and McAuley (1995a) used a small, homogeneous sample (i.e., in exercise behavior status) of fitness class participants who completed at least 8 weeks of a 12-week program. This design resulted in a highly motivated subset of participants with limited variability in motivational constructs. Courneya et al.

(2000) found social support to be a unique predictor of exercise intention and exercise stage among a large population-based Canadian sample. Although this study proposes social support should be a permanent construct for exercise prediction in the TPB, limitations of the study suggest future research is required. For example, the study used a cross-sectional design that inhibits causal implication, applied a stage measure rather than a behavior measure as suggested by the tenets of the TPB (Ajzen, 1991), and implemented a single-item measure of social support and only two items for the other TPB concepts, which are unlikely to account for the representativeness of the domains or measurement error. Further, the measurement strategy compared attitude, social support, and PBC at the global level and subjective norm at the belief level, thereby providing an inappropriate comparison of concepts. Therefore, the purpose of this study was to directly compare the utility of subjective norm versus social support for predicting exercise using a prospective design, an appropriate measurement strategy, and structural equation modeling. Besides replicating previous research with a different demographic population, this study has advantages over previous research in its prospective design and measurement off all TPB concepts and social support at the global level of abstraction. Finally, the implementation of structural equation modeling is a superior analysis over regression-path analysis because of provisions of an omnibus test of the TPB and estimates of structural effects free of error.

METHOD

Participants and Procedure

One hundred ninety-two undergraduate students participated in the study for extra credit in their introductory psychology course. The participants attended large group sessions during January and February, completing self-report measures of the TPB and social support and a 2-week follow-up measure of exercise behavior. The relatively small 2-week time lag was chosen to reflect optimal predictive accuracy, given the dynamic nature of social cognitions and the TPB tenets of time, context, target, and action (Ajzen, 1991). The mean age of participants was 19.81 years (SD = 4.05), 72.4% were women, and the mean year in university for the sample was 1.75 (SD = 1.22). Reported weekly exercise frequency over the previous month (activities for equal or greater than 30 min duration) for participants was 1.77 bouts of strenuous exercise (SD = 1.75) and 1.47 bouts of moderate exercise (SD = 1.70).

Instrument

Regular exercise was defined for all participants as activities performed at a vigorous intensity 3 or more times per week for at least 30 min each time. Participants were asked to use this definition when answering all exercise-related questions.

Exercise attitude was measured using 7-point bipolar adjective scales as suggested by Ajzen & Fishbein (1980). Although a total of eight items were measured, the hypothesized best two items that tapped the instrumental (e.g., useful-useless, wise-foolish) and affective (enjoyable-unenjoyable, pleasant-unpleasant) aspects of attitude were used to reduce the proportionality constraints in the model as suggested by Hayduk (1996). The statement that preceded the adjectives was, "For me, exercising regularly over the next 2 weeks would be. . . ." Subjective norm was measured by three items on a 7-point scale that ranged from 1 (strongly disagree) to 7 (strongly agree). The items were: (a) "Most people in my social network want me to exercise," (b) "I feel pressure to exercise from most people in my social network," and (c) "Most people in my social network think I should exercise."

Social support for exercise was measured using facets from the Social Provisions Scale (SPS; Russell & Cutrona, 1987) modified for the exercise domain by Duncan & McAuley (1993) and the Sallis Social Support for Exercise Scale (SSSES; Sallis, Grossman, Pinski, Patterson, & Nader, 1987). The SPS was developed to assess six relational provisions identified by Weiss (1974): attachment, social integration, reassurance of worth, reliable alliance, guidance, and opportunity to nurture. The degree that each provision is being met is measured using four items on a 4-point scale, ranging from completely true (4) to not at all true (1). The three provisions of reliable alliance (RA; α = .75), guidance (GU; α = .80), and social integration (SI; α = .73) were chosen as the best representative indicators of our definition of social support for exercise. The SSSES consists of 12 family and friend support items that assess the frequency of support over the past month using a 5-point scale (1 = none to 5 = very often). The family (α = .87) and friends (α = .82) subscales were both used as indicators of social support.

Perceived behavioral control was measured by three questions used by Ajzen and Madden (1986) as follows: (a) "For me, exercising regularly is . . ." on a 7-point scale ranging from 1 (extremely difficult) to 7 (extremely easy); (b) "How much control do you feel you have over exercising regularly," on a 7-point scale ranging from 1 (very little control) to 7 (complete control); (c) "How much I exercise regularly is completely up to me," on a 7-point scale ranging from 1 (strongly disagree) to 7 (strongly agree).

Exercise intention was assessed by two items as follows: (a) "I plan to participate in vigorous physical exercise at least times per week every week," rated on an open scale (Courneya, 1994); and (b) "My goal is to participate in vigorous physical exercise at least 3 times per week every week," rated on a 7-point scale from 1 (strongly disagree) to 7 (strongly agree). The loading for Indicator 1 was preset to 1.0 in the structural equation models to create a scale for Indicator 2.

Exercise behavior was measured by the Godin Leisure Time Exercise Questionnaire (Godin, Jobin, & Bouillon, 1986; Godin & Shephard, 1985). The instrument contains three open-ended questions covering the frequency of mild (e.g., easy walking), moderate (e.g., fast walking), and strenuous (e.g., jogging) exercise completed during free time for at least 30 min in a typical week. Mild and moderate exercises were excluded as indicators of exercise behavior due to their incongruence with our definition of regular exercise in the social cognitive measures. Further links to health in young and healthy populations for these intensities is tenuous (American College of Sports Medicine, 1998).

Model Specification

For specification of the latent concepts, the loading for each concept's first indicator was preset to 1.0 in the structural equation model to create a scale for the latent variable. Based on previous research identifying the proportion of error in self-reported exercise (Courneya, Estabrooks, & Nigg, 1997), the strenuous exercise indicator was given a fixed error estimate of 40% for the structural equation model.

As we hypothesized systematic error among the two affective and two instrumental attitude indicators, covariance of these errors were freed for estimation. Affective and instrumental attitudes are theorized to be conceptually distinct (i.e., possess specific variance; Ajzen & Driver, 1991), although their common variance is used for measurement (Ajzen, 1991). To account for this specific variance in our structural equation model, an a priori freeing of the correlated error for the respective affective and instrumental indicators was allowed (i.e., Affective 1 and Affective 2's error covariance and Instrumental 1 and Instrumental 2's error covariance were freed for estimation). Similarly, the correlated error for Items 2 and 3 of PBC was freed for estimation to account for any unique variance these indicators may share based on the literature suggesting that ease or difficulty and controllability may represent distinct facets of PBC (Conner & Armitage, 1998).

Structural effects of attitude, subjective norm, PBC, and intention were freed based on the tenets of the TPB (Ajzen, 1991). The structural effects of social support were freed on both exercise intention and behavior, based on the theorizing and findings of Courneya et al. (2000). Finally, the exogenous concepts of attitude, subjective norm, social support, and PBC were freed to correlate.

Assessment of Fit

The most common statistic for testing structural equation models is the chi-square (χ^2). The χ^2 goodness-of-fittest assesses the adequacy of the theorized model's creation of a covariance matrix and estimated coefficients in comparison to the observed covariance matrix. Models that result in a created covariance matrix significantly deviating from the observed covariance matrix are judged to be inadequate. For comparison of nested and alternative models, the χ^2 difference value versus degrees of freedom provides a statistical test for which model fits the observed data better.

However, the χ^2 test has been criticized as an insufficient test alone to assess model fit adequately, generally because of sample size and power estimation problems or assumptions (Hu & Bentler, 1999). Therefore, inclusion of absolute and incremental fit indexes is recommended (Hu & Bentler, 1999). Absolute fit indexes assess how well an a priori model reproduces the sample data, while incremental fit indexes measure the proportionate improvement in fit by comparing a target model with a more restricted baseline model. For the current study, root mean square error of approximation (RMSEA) was included as an absolute fit index, and the comparative fit index (CFI) was included as an index of incremental fit. General rules of thumb for acceptability of model fit using these indexes are $> .94$ for the CFI and $< .07$ for RMSEA (Hu & Bender, 1999).

Finally, when examining the significance of effects within a model, it is appropriate to use one-tailed testing if there is evidence the true population parameter estimate differs from the hypothesized population parameter estimate only in a particular direction. The TPB and social support literature in the exercise domain conceptually and statistically report positive relationships between these concepts and their criterion concepts. Therefore, a one-tailed test of significance was used for estimated structural effects and the freed error covariance within the model.

RESULTS

The variance-covariance matrix for the model was created using list-wise deletion of missing data and resulted in an analysis of 173 participants. The model was estimated with maximum likelihood procedures and assessed using LISREL 8.20 for Windows (Joreskog & Sorbom, 1997). The model suggested a moderate fit of the data with χ^2 (120, N = 173) = 165.64, p $< .05$, CFI = .97, RMSEA = .05 (see Table 1). Further, the modification indexes and standardized residuals suggested minimal changes that would significantly improve the model fit, suggesting the effects within the model can be interpreted with moderate confidence.

Table 1 details the means and standard deviations for the indicators as well as the factor loadings and error variances for the model. All loadings for the latent concepts were statistically significant (p $< .05$). Item 3 for PBC possessed the lowest loading of the model with .20; however, the correlated error for Items 2 and 3 was significant (.32, p $< .05$, one-tailed). For social support, family support had the lowest factor loading of .51, while RA possessed the strongest loading at .77. Finally, the affective and instrumental attitude items had strong factor loadings and significant correlated error (p $< .05$, one-tailed) of .10 and .25, respectively. Attitude, PBC, and social support had significant effects on intention of .10, .50, and .23, respectively (p $< .05$, one-tailed), while subjective norm was not significant (p $> .10$, one-tailed). The total explained variance of these concepts on exercise intention was 32%. Further, intention had the strongest effect on strenuous exercise behavior (.62), followed by PBC (.41), and social support (.12), with a total explained variance of 56%

TABLE 1 Factor Loadings of Social Support with the Theory of Planned Behavior

Concept	M	SD	Standardized
Attitude			
Affective 1	3.68	1.88	.91
Affective 2	3.71	1.64	.86
Instrumental 1	3.28	1.96	.85
Instrumental 2	3.15	2.18	.75
Subjective norm			
Subjective norm 1	4.77	1.72	.99
subjective norm 2	3.15	2.38	.50
Subjective norm 3	3.98	1.88	.71
Social support			
Reliable alliance	3.01	.60	.77
Guidance	3.28	.57	.68
Social integration	3.21	.54	.71
Family support	2.11	.81	.51
Friend support	2.67	.90	.74
Perceived behavioral control			
Perceived behavioral control 1	4.27	1.44	.86
Perceived behavioral control 2	5.16	1.52	.57
Perceived behavioral control 3	5.76	1.57	.20
Intention			
Intention 1	4.71	1.15	.91
Intention 2	3.23	1.48	.95
Exercise			
Strenuous	1.86	1.71	.77

Concept	Factor Loading	
	Unstandardized	Error Variance
Attitude		
Affective 1	1.00	.17★
Affective 2	.83★	.26★
Instrumental 1	.97★	.28★
Instrumental 2	.95★	.44★
Subjective norm		
Subjective norm 1	1.00	.01
subjective norm 2	.70★	.75★
Subjective norm 3	.78★	.50★
Social support		
Reliable alliance	1.00	.40★
Guidance	.84★	.54★
Social integration	.84★	.50★
Family support	.92★	.74★
Friend support	1.52★	.45★

TABLE 1 *Continued*

Concept	Unstandardized	Error Variance
Perceived behavioral control		
Perceived behavioral control 1	1.00	.27 ★
Perceived behavioral control 2	.69★	.68 ★
Perceived behavioral control 3	.25★	.96 ★
Intention		
Intention 1	1.00	.17 ★
Intention 2	1.33★	.10
Exercise		
Strenuous	1.00	.40

NOTE: M 5 mean; SD 5 standard deviation.
★ p < .05 (two-tailed) for freed estimates.

(all effects p < .05, one-tailed). The exogenous concepts were significantly correlated (p < .01, one-tailed) for PBC and subjective norm (.31), PBC and social support (.48), PBC and attitude (.19), and subjective norm and social support (.61), although attitude did not correlate significantly with subjective norm or social support (p > .10, one-tailed).

Finally, social support was tested for discriminant validity from subjective norm and PBC. This procedure was performed to ascertain whether social support is a distinct predictor of exercise intention from subjective norm and PBC. Concept distinction was achieved by constraining the correlations of social support and subjective norm, or social support and PBC to unity, and then comparing this χ^2 to a χ^2 estimated as two correlated concepts (Anderson & Gerbing, 1988). Models consisting of correlated concepts for social support and subjective norm and social support and PBC proved a significantly better fit than models with the correlations constrained to unity with χ^2 difference (1) = 24.88, p χ^2 .01, and χ^2 difference (1) = 27.85, p χ^2 .01, respectively. As such, social support was found to possess discriminant validity from both subjective norm and PBC.

DISCUSSION

The purpose of this study was to compare the relative value of social support and subjective norm for predicting exercise intention and behavior within the theory of planned behavior. We extended previous research on this topic by using a prospective design, validated measures of social support and subjective norm, and structural equation modeling. Overall, the model we tested suggested a moderate fit of the data, implying the effects within the model can be interpreted with moderate confidence. Equally important, social support was found to possess discriminant validity from both subjective norm and PBC, supporting the inclusion of social support within the TPB as a distinct concept (cf. Courneya & McAuley, 1995b).

One key finding of the present study was that social support had a significant effect on intention along with PBC and attitude. This suggests that individuals are influenced by perceived support for exercise when forming exercise intentions independent of attitudes, subjective norms, and perceptions of behavioral control. This finding supports the research by Courneya et al. (2000) and suggests that social support may be superior to subjective norm for understanding exercise intentions. Consequently, replacing subjective norm with social support should receive consideration when applying the TPB to exercise.

A second key finding of this study identified social support to exert a significant direct effect on strenuous exercise behavior while controlling for the significant effects of intention and PBC. This finding supports the research and theorizing by Courneya et al. (2000) suggesting that exercise behavior, not being under complete volitional control, is influenced by assistance from others (i.e., social support). This direct effect on strenuous exercise behavior may be explained to the extent that social support is a reflection of the actual amount of social support received. That social support was significant even when controlling for PBC and intention further advocates for the inclusion of social support within the TPB in the exercise domain. Few constructs have shown this predictive utility with the exception of past behavior.

The practical implication of this study suggests that interventions targeting social support would improve exercise intentions and subsequent behavior independent of interventions targeting behavioral, normative and control beliefs that make up the TPB constructs of attitude, subjective norms, and PBG respectively. As the study also found that social support predicted intention superior to attitude and subjective norm, social support-based interventions may most effectively influence exercise intentions after PBC.

Investigating the social support concept in the model found that perceiving a reliable alliance (e.g., someone to depend on for motivation when needed) with at least one person for exercise support was the most important indicator of the social support construct, with 59% of its variance explained. In contrast, family social support was the poorest indicator in this sample, sharing only 26% of the variance in the overall social support concept. Still, family social support was a significant indicator and may simply represent the importance of friend over family social support among college-aged individuals. Future research is required among other populations to verify this possibility.

Limitations to the preceding study may confine the generalizability of these findings, and, therefore, warrant mentioning. First, the present study uses a convenience sample of university undergraduates and self-reported exercise behavior. Future research would benefit by using more objective measures of exercise (e.g., attendance to a fitness facility) and diverse samples of multiple age groups or clinical populations to strengthen the cross-validation and theoretical veracity of the findings. Second, although the social support construct was significant in the TPB model, it lacked the specific measurement characteristics of action, target, context, and time outlined by the TPB (Ajzen, 1991). As such, future research may even improve on these findings further by including a social support measure that follows the measurement specifications outlined in the TPB (Courneya et al., 2000).

REFERENCES

Ajzen, I. (1991). The theory of planned behavior. *Organizational Behavior and Human Decision Processes,* 50, 179–211.

Ajzen, I., & Driver, B. L. (1991). Prediction of leisure participation from behavioral, normative, and control beliefs: An application of the theory of planned behavior. *Leisure Sciences,* 13, 185–204.

Ajzen, I., & Fishbein, M. (1980). *Understanding attitudes and predicting social behavior.* Englewood Cliffs, NJ: Prentice-Hall.

Ajzen, I., & Madden, T. J. (1986). Prediction of goal-directed behavior: Attitude, intentions, and perceived behavioral control. *Journal of Experimental Social Psychology,* 22, 453–474.

American College of Sports Medicine. (1998). Position stand on the recommended quantity and quality of exercise for developing and maintaining cardiorespiratory and muscular fitness and flexibility in adults. *Medicine and Science in Sports and Exercise,* 30, 975–991.

Anderson, J. C., & Gerbing, D. W. (1988). Structural equation, modeling in practice: A review and recommended two-step approach. *Psychological Bulletin,* 103, 411–423.

Conner, M., & Armitage, C.J. (1998). Extending the theory of planned behavior: A review and avenues for further research. *Journal of Applied Social Psychology,* 28, 1429–1464.

Courneya, K. S. (1994). Predicting repeated behavior from intention: The issue of scale correspondence. *Journal of Applied Social Psychology,* 24, 580–594.

Courneya, K. S., Estabrooks, P. A., & Nigg, C. R. (1997). A simple reinforcement strategy for increasing attendance at a fitness facility. *Health Education & Behavior,* 24, 708–715.

Courneya, K. S., & McAuley, E. (1995a). Cognitive mediators of the social influence exercise adherence relationship: A test of the theory of planned behavior. *Journal of Behavioral Medicine,* 18, 499–515.

Courneya, K. S., & McAuley, E. (1995b). Reliability and discriminant validity of subjective norm, social support, and cohesion in an exercise setting. *Journal of Sport and Exercise Psychology,* 17, 499–515.

Courneya, K. S., Plotnikoff, R. C., Hotz, S. B., & Birkett, N.J. (2000) Social support and the theory of planned behavior in the exercise domain. *American Journal of Health Behavior,* 24, 300–308.

Duncan, T. E., & McAuley, E. (1993). Social support and efficacy cognitions in exercise adherence: A latent growth curve analysis. *Journal of Behavioral Medicine,* 16, 199–218.

Godin, G., & Kok, G. (1996). The theory of planned behavior: A review of its applications to health-related behaviors. *American Journal of Health Promotion,* 11, 87–98.

Godin, G., Jobin, J., & Bouillon, J. (1986). Assessment of leisure time exercise behavior by self-report: A concurrent validity study. *Canadian Journal of Public Health,* 77, 359–361.

Godin, G., & Shephard, R.J. (1985). A simple method to assess exercise behavior in the community. *Canadian Journal of Applied Sport Science,* 10, 141–146.

Hausenblaus, H. A., Carron, A. V., & Mack, D. E. (1997). Application of the theories of reasoned action and planned behavior to exercise behavior: A meta-analysis. *Journal of Sport & Exercise Psychology,* 19, 36–51.

Hayduk, L. A. (1996). *LISREL Issues, Debates, and Strategies.* Baltimore: Johns Hopkins University Press.

Hu, L., & Bentler, P.M. (1999). Cuttoff Criteria for fit indices in covariance structure analysis: Conventional criteria versus new alternatives. *Structural Equation Modeling,* 6, 1–55.

Joreskog, K., & Sorbom, D. (1997). *LISREL 8.20 for Windows.* Chicago: Scientific Software International Inc.

Russell, D., & Cutrona, C. E. (1987). The provisions of social relationships and adaptation to stress. *Advances in Personal Relationships,* 1, 37–67.

Sallis, J. F., Grossman, M. S., Pinski, R. B., Patterson, T. L., & Nader, P. R. (1987). The development of scales to measure social support for diet and exercise behaviors. *American Journal of Epidemiology,* 127, 933–941.

Weiss, R. S. (1974). The provisions of social relationships. In Z. Rubin (Ed.), *Doing Unto Others* (pp. 17–26). Englewood Cliffs, NJ: Prentice Hall.

DISCUSSION QUESTIONS

1. What is the purpose of this study?
2. How did the authors define "regular exercise"?
3. What did the researchers find?
4. What are the practical implications of this study?

4

A "Stages of Change" Approach to Helping Patients Change Behavior

Gretchen L. Zimmerman, Cynthia G. Olsen, and Michael F. Bosworth

Helping patients change behavior is an important role for family physicians. Change interventions are especially useful in addressing lifestyle modification for disease prevention, long-term disease management and addictions. The concepts of "patient noncompliance" and motivation often focus on patient failure. Understanding patient readiness to make change, appreciating barriers to change and helping patients anticipate relapse can improve patient satisfaction and lower physician frustration during the change process. In this article, we review the Transtheoretical Model of Change, also known as the Stages of Change model, and discuss its application to the family practice setting. The Readiness to Change Ruler and the Agenda-Setting Chart are two simple tools that can be used in the office to promote discussion. (Am Fam Physician 2000; 61:1409–16.)

One role of family physicians is to assist patients in understanding their health and to help them make the changes necessary for health improvement. Exercise programs, stress management techniques and dietary restrictions represent some common interventions that require patient motivation. A change in patient lifestyle is necessary for successful management of long-term illness, and relapse can often be attributed to lapses in healthy behavior by the patient. Patients easily understand lifestyle

American Family Physician, March 1, 2000 v61 i5 p1409
"A 'Stages of Change' Approach to Helping Patients Change Behavior" by Gretchen L. Zimmerman, Cynthia G. Olsen, and Michael F. Bosworth. © 2000 American Academy of Family Physicians

modifications (i.e., "I need to reduce the fat in my diet in order to control my weight.") but consistent, life-long behavior changes are difficult.

Much has been written about success and failure rates in helping patients change, about barriers to change and about the role of physicians in improving patient outcomes. Recommendations for physicians helping patients to change have ranged from the "just do it" approach to suggesting extended office visits, often incorporating behavior modification, record-keeping suggestions and follow-up telephone calls.(1–3) Repeatedly educating the patient is not always successful and can become frustrating for the physician and patient. Furthermore, promising patients an improved outcome does not guarantee their motivation for long-term change. Patients may view physicians who use a confrontational approach as being critical rather than supportive. Relapse during any treatment program is sometimes viewed as a failure by the patient and the physician. A feeling of failure, especially when repeated, may cause patients to give up and avoid contact with their physician or avoid treatment altogether. After physicians invest time and energy in promoting change, patients who fail are often labeled "noncompliant" or "unmotivated." Labeling a patient in this way places responsibility for failure on the patient's character and ignores the complexity of the behavior change process.

LESSONS LEARNED FROM SMOKING AND ALCOHOL CESSATION

Research into smoking cessation and alcohol abuse has advanced our understanding of the change process, giving us new directions for health promotion. Current views depict patients as being in a process of change; when physicians choose a mode of intervention, "one size doesn't fit all."(4,5) Two important developments include the Stages of Change model(4) and motivational interviewing strategies.(6) The developers of the Stages of Change model used factor and cluster analytic methods in retrospective, prospective and cross-sectional studies of the ways people quit smoking. The model has been validated and applied to a variety of behaviors that include smoking cessation, exercise behavior, contraceptive use and dietary behavior.(7–10) Simple and effective "stage-based" approaches derived from the Stages of Change model(4) demonstrate widespread utility.(11–16) In addition, brief counseling sessions (lasting five to 15 minutes) have been as effective as longer visits.(17,18)

UNDERSTANDING CHANGE

Physicians should remember that behavior change is rarely a discrete, single event. Physicians sometimes see patients who, after experiencing a medical crisis and being advised to change the contributing behavior, readily comply. More often, physicians encounter patients who seem unable or unwilling to change. During the past decade, behavior change has come to be understood as a process of identifiable stages through which patients pass. Physicians can enhance those stages by taking specific action. Understanding this process provides physicians with additional tools to assist patients, who are often as discouraged as their physicians with their lack of change.

The Stages of Change model(4) shows that, for most persons, a change in behavior occurs gradually, with the patient moving from being uninterested, unaware or unwilling to make a change (precontemplation), to considering a change (contemplation), to deciding and preparing to make a change. Genuine, determined action is then taken and, over time, attempts to maintain the new behavior occur. Relapses are almost inevitable and become part of the process of working toward life-long change.

Precontemplation Stage

During the precontemplation stage, patients do not even consider changing. Smokers who are "in denial" may not see that the advice applies to them personally. Patients with high cholesterol levels may feel "immune" to the health problems that strike others. Obese patients may have tried unsuccessfully so many times to lose weight that they have simply given up.

Contemplation Stage

During the contemplation stage, patients are ambivalent about changing. Giving up an enjoyed behavior causes them to feel a sense of loss despite the perceived gain. During this stage, patients assess barriers (e.g., time, expense, hassle, fear, "I know I need to, doc, but . . .") as well as the benefits of change.

Preparation Stage

During the preparation stage, patients prepare to make a specific change. They may experiment with small changes as their determination to change increases. For example, sampling low-fat foods may be an experimentation with or a move toward greater dietary modification. Switching to a different brand of cigarettes or decreasing their drinking signals that they have decided a change is needed.

Action Stage

The action stage is the one that most physicians are eager to see their patients reach. Many failed New Year's resolutions provide evidence that if the prior stages have been glossed over, action itself is often not enough. Any action taken by patients should be praised because it demonstrates the desire for lifestyle change.

MAINTENANCE AND RELAPSE PREVENTION

Maintenance and relapse prevention involve incorporating the new behavior "over the long haul." Discouragement over occasional "slips" may halt the change process and result in the patient giving up. However, most patients find themselves "recycling" through the stages of change several times before the change becomes truly established.

The Stages of Change model(4) encompasses many concepts from previously developed models. The Health Belief model,(19) the Locus of Control model(20) and behavioral models fit together well within this framework. During the precontemplation stage, patients do not consider change. They may not believe that their behavior is a problem or that it will negatively affect them (Health Belief Model [19]), or they may be resigned to their unhealthy behavior because of previous failed efforts and no longer believe that they have control (external Locus of Control[20]). During the contemplation stage, patients struggle with ambivalence, weighing the pros and cons of their current behavior and the benefits of and barriers to change (Health Belief Model[19]). Cognitive-behavioral models of change (e.g., focusing on coping skills or environmental manipulation) and 12-Step programs fit well in the preparation, action and maintenance stages (Table 1).(4,6)

TABLE 1   Stages of Change Model

Stage in Transtheoretical Model of Change	Patient Stage
Precontemplation	Not thinking about change
	May be resigned
	Feeling of no control
	Denial: does not believe it applies to self
	Believes consequences are not serious
Contemplation	Weighing benefits and costs of behavior proposed change
Preparation	Experimenting with small changes
Action	Taking a definitive action to change
Maintenance	Maintaining new behavior over time
Relapse	Experiencing normal part of process of change
	Usually feels demoralized

Stage in Transtheoretical Model of Change	Incorporating Other Explanatory/Treatment Models
Precontemplation	Locus of Control
	Health Belief Model
	Motivational interviewing
Contemplation	Health Belief Model
	Motivational interviewing
Preparation	Cognitive-behavioral therapy
Action	Cognitive-behavioral therapy
	12-Step program
Maintenance	Cognitive-behavioral therapy
	12-Step program
Relapse	Motivational interviewing
	12-Step program

Information from Prochaska JO, DiClemente CC, Norcross JC. In search of how people change. *Am Psychol* 1992;47:1102–4, and Miller WR, Rollnick S. *Motivational interviewing: Preparing people to change addictive behavior.* New York: Guilford, 1991:191–202.

INTERVENTIONS

The Stages of Change model(4) is useful for selecting appropriate interventions. By identifying a patient's position in the change process, physicians can tailor the intervention, usually with skills they already possess. Thus, the focus of the office visit is not to convince the patient to change behavior but to help the patient move along the stages of change. Using the framework of the Stages of Change model,(4) the goal for a single encounter is a shift from the grandiose ("Get patient to change unhealthy behavior.") to the realistic ("Identify the stage of change and engage patient in a process to move to the next stage.").(4)

Starting with brief and simple advice makes sense because some patients will indeed change their behavior at the directive of their physician. (This step also prevents precontemplators from rationalizing that, "My doctor never told me to quit.") Rather than viewing this step as the intervention, physicians should view this as the opening assessment of where patients are in the behavior change process. A patient's response to this direct advice will provide helpful information on which physicians can base the next step in the physician-patient dialog. Rather than continue merely to educate and admonish, interventions based on the Stages of Change model(4) can be appropriately tailored to each patient to enhance success. A physician who provides concrete advice about smoking cessation when a patient remarks that family members who smoke have not died from lung cancer has not matched the intervention to the patient's stage of change. A few minutes spent listening to the patient and then appropriately matching physician intervention to patient readiness to change can improve communication and outcome.

Patients at the precontemplation and contemplation stages can be especially challenging for physicians. Motivational interviewing techniques have been found to be most effective. Miller and colleagues(21) replicated studies with "problem drinkers," demonstrating that an empathetic therapist style was predictive of decreased drinking while a confrontational style predicted increased drinking. Motivational interviewing incorporates empathy and reflective listening with key questions so that physicians are simultaneously patient-centered and directive. Controlled studies have shown motivational interviewing techniques to be at least as effective as cognitive-behavioral techniques and 12-step facilitation interventions, and they are easily adaptable for use by family physicians.(22–27)

HELPING THE "STUCK" PATIENT

The goal for patients at the precontemplation stage is to begin to think about changing a behavior. The task for physicians is to empathetically engage patients in contemplating change (Table 2).(6) During this stage, patients appear argumentative, hopeless or in "denial," and the natural tendency is for physicians to try to "convince" them, which usually engenders resistance.

TABLE 2   The Stages of Change and Opportunities for Physician Intervention

Precontemplation stage

Goal: patient will begin thinking about change.

Use relationship-building skills.

Personalize risk factors.

Give data about the patient's vitals, laboratory results, etc., compared with the norm.

Rather than using scare tactics, express your caring concern.

Use teachable moments (the symptom as a message).

Educate in small bits, repeatedly, over time.

Ask "How would you know if your _____ was a problem for you?"

Ask "If you were to decide to change, what do you imagine might be some advantages?"

Contemplation stage

Goal: patient will examine benefits and barriers to change.

Elicit from the patient reasons to change and the consequences of not changing.

Explore ambivalence; praise the patient for considering the difficulties of change.

Restate both sides of ambivalence.

Question possible solutions for one barrier at a time.

Pose advice gently as "a solution that has been effective for some patients and might be adaptable to you" to avoid patient's natural resistance.

Preparation stage

Goal: patient will discover elements necessary for decisive action.

Encourage the patient's efforts.

Ask which strategies the patient has decided on for risk situations.

Ask for a change date.

Action stage

Goal: patient will take decisive action.

Reinforce the decision.

Delight in even small successes.

View problems as helpful information.

Ask what else is needed for success.

Maintenance stage

Goal: patient will incorporate change into daily lifestyle.

Continue reinforcement.

Ask what strategies have been helpful and what situations problematic (provides physician with more information to use with other patients as well).

Relapse stage

Goal: learn from the temporary success and re-engage patient in the change process.

Reframe from "failure" to "successful for a while plus new lessons" for continued success.

Remind the patient that change is a process, that most people "recycle."

Adapted with permission from Miller WR, Rollnick S. *Motivational interviewing: preparing people to change addictive behavior.* New York: Guilford, 1991:191–202.

Patient resistance is evidence that the physician has moved too far ahead of the patient in the change process, and a shift back to empathy and thought-provoking questions is required. Physicians can engage patients in the contemplation process by developing and maintaining a positive relationship, personalizing risk factors and posing questions that provoke thoughts about patient risk factors and the perceived "bottom line."

The wording of questions and the patient's style of "not thinking about changing" are also important. As precontemplators respond to questions, rather than jumping in and providing advice or appearing judgmental, the task for physicians is to reflect with empathy, instill hope and gently point out discrepancies between goals and statements. Asking argumentative patients, "Do you want to die from this?" may be perceived as a threat and can elicit more resistance and hostility. On the other hand, asking patients, "How will you know that it's time to quit?" allows patients to be their "own expert" and can help them begin a thought process that extends beyond the examination room. Well-phrased questions will leave patients pondering the answers that are right for them and will move them along the process of change (Table 3).(6)

It is not unusual for some patients to spend years in the contemplation stage, which physicians can easily recognize by their "yes, but" statements. Empathy, validation, praise and encouragement are necessary during all stages but especially when patients struggle with ambivalence and doubt their ability

---

TABLE 3   Questions for Patients in the Precontemplation and Contemplation Stages[*]

Precontemplation stage
    Goal: patient will begin thinking about change.
    "What would have to happen for you to know that this is a problem?"
    "What warning signs would let you know that this is a problem?"
    "Have you tried to change in the past?"

Contemplation stage
    Goal: patient will examine benefits and barriers to change.
    "Why do you want to change at this time?"
    "What were the reasons for not changing?"
    "What would keep you from changing at this time?"
    "What are the barriers today that keep you from change?"
    "What might help you with that aspect?"
    "What things (people, programs and behaviors) have helped in the past?"
    "What would help you at this time?"
    "What do you think you need to learn about changing?"

[*]—The change can be applied to any desirable behavior (e.g., smoking or drinking cessation, losing weight, exercise).

Information from Miller WR, Rollnick S. *Motivational interviewing: Preparing people to change addictive behavior.* NewYork: Guilford, 1991:191–202.

to accomplish the change. Physicians may find statements such as the following to be useful: "Yes, it is difficult. What difficult things have you accomplished in the past?" or "I've seen you handle some tough stuff, I know you'll be able to conquer this." A successful approach calls for physicians to ask patients about possible strategies to overcome barriers and then arrive at a commitment to pursue one strategy before the next visit. It is also productive to ask patients about their previous methods and attempts to change behavior. Barriers and gaps in patients' knowledge can then surface for further discussion.

When patients experiment with changing a behavior (preparation stage) such as cutting down on smoking or starting to exercise, they are shifting into more decisive action. Physicians should encourage them to address the barriers to full-fledged action. While continuing to explore patient ambivalence, strategies should shift from motivational to behavioral skills. During the action and maintenance stages, physicians should continue to ask about successes and difficulties—and be generous with praise and admiration.

RELAPSE FROM CHANGED BEHAVIOR

Relapse is common during lifestyle changes. Physicians can help by explaining to patients that even though a relapse has occurred, they have learned something new about themselves and about the process of changing behavior. For example, patients who previously stopped smoking may have learned that it is best to avoid smoke-filled environments. Patients with diabetes who are on a restricted diet may learn that they can be successful in adhering to the diet if they order from a menu rather than choose the all-you-can-eat buffet. Focusing on the successful part of the plan ("You did it for six days; what made that work?") shifts the focus from failure, promotes problem solving and offers encouragement. The goal here is to support patients and re-engage their efforts in the change process. They should be left with a sense of realistic goals to prevent discouragement, and their positive steps toward behavior change should be acknowledged.(24)

ADDITIONAL TOOLS

Two techniques useful in the primary care setting are the Readiness to Change Ruler and the Agenda-Setting Chart.(26,27) The Readiness to Change Ruler, which is incorporated in Figure 1,(4,26,27) is a simple, straight line drawn on a paper that represents a continuum from the left "not prepared to change" to the right "ready to change." Patients are asked to mark on the line their current position in the change process. Physicians should then question patients about why they did not place the mark further to the left (which elicits motivational statements) and what it would take to move the line further to the right (which

FIGURE 1. The Readiness to Change Ruler can be used with patients contemplating any desirable behavior, such as smoking cessation, losing weight, exercise or substance-abuse cessation. Information from references 4, 26 and 27.

Changing Behavior for Your Health

1. On the line below, mark where you are now on this line that measures change in behavior. Are you not prepared to change, already changing or someplace in the middle?

   Not prepared to change   Already changing

2. Answer the questions below that apply to you.
   - If your mark is on the left side of the line:
     How will you know when it's time to think about changing?
     What signals will tell you to start thinking about changing?
     What qualities in yourself are important to you?
     What connection is there between those qualities and "not considering a change"?
   - If your mark is somewhere in the middle:
     Why did you put your mark there and not further to the left?
     What might make you put your mark a little further to the right?
     What are the good things about the way you're currently trying to change?
     What are the not-so-good things?
     What would be the good result of changing?
     What are the barriers to changing?
   - If your mark is on the right side of the line:
     Pick one of the barriers to change and list some things that could help you overcome this barrier.
     Pick one of those things that could help and decide to do it by
     _____ (write in a specific date).
   - If you've taken a serious step in making a change:
     What made you decide on that particular step?
     What has worked in taking this step?
     What helped it work?
     What could help it work even better?
     What else would help?
     Can you break that helpful step down into smaller pieces?
     Pick one of those pieces and decide to do it by _____ (write in a specific date).
   - If you're changing and trying to maintain that change:
     Congratulations! What's helping you?
     What else would help?
     What are your high-risk situations?
   - If you've "fallen off the wagon":
     What worked for a while?
     Don't kick yourself—long-term change almost always takes a few cycles.
     What did you learn from the experience that will help you when you give it another try?

3. The following are stages people go through in making important changes in their health behaviors. All the stages are important. We learn from each stage.

   We go **from** "not thinking about it" **to** "weighing the pros and cons" **to** "making little changes and figuring out how to deal with the real hard parts" **to** "doing it!" **to** "making it part of our lives."

   Many people "fall off the wagon" and go through all the stages several times before the change really lasts.

elicits perceived barriers). Physicians can ask patients for suggestions about ways to overcome an identified barrier and actions that might be taken before the next visit.

The Agenda-Setting Chart is useful when multiple lifestyle changes are recommended for long-term disease management (e.g., diabetes or prevention of heart disease). The physician draws multiple circles on a paper, filling in behavior changes that have been shown to affect the disease in question and adding a few blank circles. For example, "lose weight," "stop smoking" and "exercise" may each occupy a circle—all of them representing behavior changes that are known to reduce the risk of heart disease. The physician begins the patient session with, "Let's spend a few minutes talking about some of the ways we can work together to improve your health. In the circles are some factors we can tackle to improve your health. Are there other factors that you know would be important to address that we should add to the blank circles?" Discussion then revolves around the patient's priority area and identifies a goal that might be achievable before the next office visit.

INVOLVING OTHERS

While no research is available that uses the Stages of Change model(4) in teaching families how to intervene with their loved one's health-risk behavior, training about this model may help family members view the situation differently. Physicians can enlist the help of other health care professionals (e.g., nutritionists, nurses, mental health personnel) to reinforce the message that a change in behavior is needed and to provide additional education and skill information to the patient. Referral can also reduce some patient care burden for physicians. Physicians should document the content and outcome of patient conversations, including specific tasks and plans for follow-up.

FINAL COMMENT

Family physicians need to develop techniques to assist patients who will benefit from behavior change. Traditional advice and patient education does not work with all patients. Understanding the stages through which patients pass during the process of successfully changing a behavior enables physicians to tailor interventions individually. These methods can be applied to many areas of health changing behavior.

REFERENCES

1. Miller NH, Smith PM, DeBusk RF, Sobel DS, Taylor CB. Smoking cessation in hospitalized patients. *Arch Intern Med* 1997;157:409–15.
2. Kahan M, Wilson L, Becker L. Effectiveness of physician-based interventions with problem drinkers: a review. *CMAJ* 1995;152:851–9.

3. Glynn TJ, Manley MW. *How to help your patients stop smoking: a National Cancer Institute Manual for Physicians.* U.S. Department of Health and Human Services, Public Health Service, National Institutes of Health, National Cancer Institute, Division of Cancer Prevention and Control. NIH publication no. 95–3064;1995.

4. Prochaska JO, DiClemente CC, Norcross JC. In search of how people change. *Am Psychol* 1992; 47:1102–4.

5. Miller WR. What really drives change? *Addiction* 1993;88:1479–80.

6. Miller WR, Rollnick S. *Motivational interviewing: preparing people to change addictive behavior.* New York: Guilford, 1991.

7. Prochaska JO, Velicer WF, Rossi JS, Goldstein MG, Marcus BH, Rakowski W, et al. Stages of change and decisional balance for 12 problem behaviors. *Health Psychol* 1994;13:39–46.

8. Grimley DM, Riley GE, Bellis JM, Prochaska JO. Assessing the stages of change and decision-making for contraceptive use for the prevention of pregnancy, sexually transmitted diseases, and acquired immunodeficiency syndrome. *Health Educ Q* 1993;29:455–70.

9. Hellman EA. Use of the stages of change in exercise adherence model among older adults with a cardiac diagnosis. *J Cardiopulm Rehabil* 1997;17:145–55.

10. Glanz K, Patterson RE, Kristal AR, DiClemente CC, Heimendinger J, Linnan L, et al. Stages of change in adopting healthy diets: fat, fiber, and correlates of nutrient intake. *Health Educ Q* 1994;21:499–519.

11. Hughes JR. An algorithm for smoking cessation. *Arch Fam Med* 1994;3:280–5.

12. Barnes HN, Samet JH. Brief interventions with substance-abusing patients. Med Clin North Am 1997;81:867–79.

13. Campbell MK, DeVellis BM, Strecher VJ, Ammerman AS, DeVellis RF, Sandler RS. Improving dietary behavior: the effectiveness of tailored messages in primary care settings. *Am J Public Health* 1994; 84:783–7.

14. Calfas KJ, Sallis JF, Oldenburg B, French M. Mediators of change in physical activity following an intervention in primary care: PACE. *Prev Med* 1997;26:297–304.

15. Weinstein ND, Lyon JE, Sandman PM, Cuite CL. Experimental evidence for stages of health behavior change: the precaution adoption process model applied to home radon testing. *Health Psychol* 1998;17:445–53.

16. Cabral RJ, Galavotti C, Gargiullo PM, Armstrong K, Cohen A, Gielen AC, et al. Paraprofessional delivery of a theory based HIV prevention counseling intervention for women. *Public Health Rep* 1996: 111(suppl 1):75–82.

17. A cross-national trial of brief interventions with heavy drinkers. WHO Brief Intervention Study Group. *Am J Public Health* 1996;86:948–55.

18. Oliansky DM, Wildenhaus KJ, Manlove K, Arnold T, Schoener EP. Effectiveness of brief interventions in reducing substance use among at-risk primary care patients in three community-based clinics. *Substance Abuse* 1997;18:95–103.

19. Janz NK, Becker MH. The Health Belief Model: a decade later. *Health Educ Q* 1984;11:1–47.

20. Rotter JB. Generalized expectancies of internal versus external control of reinforcement. *Psychol Monogr* 1966;80:1–28.

21. Miller WR, Benefield RG, Tonigan JS. Enhancing motivation for change in problem drinking: a controlled comparison of two therapist styles. *J Consult Clin Psychol* 1993;61:455–61.

22. Australian Medical and Professional Society on Alcohol and Other Drugs. *Drug and alcohol review.* Abingdon, United Kingdom: Abingdon Carfax, 1996.

23. Matching alcoholism treatments to client heterogeneity: project MATCH posttreatment drinking outcomes. Project Match Research Group. *J Stud Alcohol* 1997;58:7–29.

24. Smith DE, Heckemeyer CM, Kratt PP, Mason DA. Motivational interviewing to improve adherence to a behavioral weight-control program for older obese women with NIDDM. A pilot study. *Diabetes Care* 1997;20:52–4.

25. Rollnick S, Butler CC, Stott NC. Helping smokers make decisions: the enhancement of brief intervention for general medical practice. *Patient Educ Couns* 1997;31:191–203.

26. Miller WR, Rollnick W. Motivational interviewing: preparing people to change. Professional training videotape series. Albuquerque, N.M.: University of New Mexico, 1998.

27. Stott NC, Rees M, Rollnick S, Pill RM, Hackett P. Professional responses to innovation in clinical method: diabetes care and negotiating skills. *Patient Educ Couns* 1996;29:67–73.

DISCUSSION QUESTIONS

1. What is one lesson that researchers have learned from smoking and alcohol cessation programs?

2. What are the 4 stages of change? Explain how a patient would behave in each stage.

3. Why is the "Stage of Change" model useful for physicians?

4. According to this model, why does patient resistance occur?

5. How could a physician turn a relapse (a negative event) into a learning opportunity for the patient?

6. Do you personally think the "Stage of Change" model would be a useful tool for physicians to use? Why or why not?

5

Adolescents React to the Events of September 11, 2001: Focused Versus Ambient Impact

Carol K. Whalen, Barbara Henker, Pamela S. King, Larry
D. Jamner, and Linda Levine

INTRODUCTION

At first I was very stunned. I couldn't believe all that was happening. But the next couple of weeks I was seriously depressed. I stayed up late each night online wanting to feel connected and sharing with my friends all we thought of the 9/11 events. I wore black the whole week and attended prayer services. But I still think of those people who we'll never get the chance to meet.

(Female high school senior, age 17)

Little is known about normative affective reactions to nonnormative events. The bulk of the burgeoning literature on disasters focuses on posttraumatic stress symptoms and disorders in people who were in close proximity to a disaster, many of whom experienced major injuries and loss. Much less is known

Journal of Abnormal Child Psychology, Feb 2004 v32 i1 p1(11)
"Adolescents React to the Events of September 11, 2001: Focused Versus Ambient Impact" by Carol K. Whalen, Barbara Henker, Pamela S. King, Larry D. Jamner, and Linda Levine. © 2004 Plenum Publishing Corporation

about long-distance effects on everyday functioning. Because of the immediacy, breadth, and repetitiveness of media coverage in contemporary society, events that were previously experienced as local crises, such as mining accidents or child kidnappings, rapidly develop into national tragedies. Thus it seems critical to gain an understanding of the impact of distant traumas on psychological health and everyday functioning.

Exposure-Response Relationships and Predisaster Functioning

Not surprisingly, people who experience serious loss, disruption, injury, or death of a loved one following a traumatic event tend to show more severe psychological distress than do those who suffer fewer consequences (Katz, Pellegrino, Pandya, Ng, & DeLisi, 2002; Pfefferbaum, 1997; Yule, Perrin, & Smith, 2001). An exposure-response gradient appears to apply not only to extent of personal loss, but also to degree of proximity, as illustrated by Pynoos and colleagues' report (Pynoos, Nader, Frederick, Gonda, & Stuber, 1987) of an association between the number of posttraumatic stress disorder (PTSD) symptoms and the distance the child was from a fatal sniper attack on a schoolyard. The degree to which rapid and repetitive media coverage may be leveling this proximity gradient is an important question.

The few studies conducted prior to September 11 of "distant traumas," catastrophic events in which the individual is not directly involved, document reactions ranging from mild to severe and from brief to enduring. Terr et al. (1999) found unsalutary effects of the *Challenger* spacecraft explosion on young people at two levels of exposure, close (East Coast) versus distant (West Coast). As expected, the East Coast youngsters appeared more symptomatic. Although many of the problems and PTSD symptoms diminished over the course of a year, negative views about institutions and pessimistic expectations for the world's future remained stable or increased over time, especially among adolescents (Terr et al., 1997). These studies provide an important perspective, demonstrating that young people are affected not only by personal traumas, but also by more remote disasters, and that some of these effects may persist.

Another important dimension, in addition to degree of exposure, is predisaster functioning (Katz et al., 2002; Yule et al., 2001). People with similar levels of exposure show dissimilar reactions, some experiencing difficulties and others demonstrating resilience. Prospective studies of disaster reactions are needed so that risk and protective factors can be identified and cost-effective intervention strategies developed. One of the most robust findings that has surfaced from the few studies that included predisaster information is a link between preexisting anxiety levels and both the intensity and duration of postdisaster difficulties (Asarnow et al., 1999; La Greca, Silverman, & Wasserstein, 1998).

The Attacks of September 11, 2001

There are several ways in which the attacks of September 11, 2001, differ from the panoply of natural and human-generated disasters studied to date. One of the most obvious is the number of people killed and the even larger numbers who suffered severe losses and major life changes. Another difference is that most disasters are relatively discrete events: The *Challenger* explosion happened in moments, as did the Oklahoma City bombing, and the shootings at Columbine High School. In contrast, the undoubtedly unique attacks of September 11 have been associated with extensive and enduring threats, including sustained military action, anthrax infections and warnings of bioterrorism, and highly publicized alerts predicting repeated attacks and counseling heightened vigilance. In many ways, September 11 is not over; one cannot yet identify a point at which the September 11 disaster ends and the recovery begins. For these reasons, the psychological effects of the attacks and their aftermath might be expected to be both more pervasive and more enduring than those of other recent tragedies.

Studies published during the first year following the attacks have reported widespread effects on people in close proximity as well as those more distant from the disaster sites (Galea et al., 2002). In a study of over 3,500 adults residing in New York, New Jersey, or Connecticut, it was found that nearly half reported anger after the attacks and significant numbers of them increased consumption of alcohol and cigarettes (Centers for Disease Control and Prevention, 2002). A nationwide telephone survey revealed that 44% of adults suffered marked stress reactions immediately after the events of September 11, 2001; according to parent report, 35% of children age 5 or older showed stress symptoms such as trouble concentrating, and 47% worried about their safety (Schuster et al., 2001). Silver, Holman, McIntosh, Poulin, and Gil-Rivas (2002) found that 17% of a nationwide sample of adults residing outside of New York City reported posttraumatic stress symptoms at 2 months and nearly 6% reported symptoms at 6 months. Significant predictors included not only severity of exposure and demographic variables such as gender and marital status, but also coping styles such as behavioral disengagement and self-blame, a finding that replicates results from a study of children exposed to Hurricane Andrew (Vernberg, La Greca, Silverman, & Prinstein, 1996). Especially noteworthy is the fact that reactions may extend far beyond the terrorist acts themselves, as demonstrated by Halpern-Felsher and Millstein's (2002) finding that adolescents indicated increased perceptions of vulnerability to death from a tornado, an earthquake, or any cause following the September 11 attacks.

Focused Versus Ambient Impact

Most studies of the psychological effects of major disasters and tragedies, including those assessing the consequences of September 11, examine what might be called focused impact. Questions were framed within the context of the disaster, and people were asked how their thoughts, feelings, or behaviors have been affected. More difficult to assess is the more diffuse, ambient impact, changes in daily functioning that are not attributed explicitly to the disaster and may not even be recognized by people experiencing the changes. Focused impact is more directed or targeted, whereas ambient impact is more subtle and possibly also more pervasive and insidious. From a cognitive processing perspective, focused impact involves relative judgments, before–after comparisons, similar to a "cued recall" paradigm. In contrast, ambient impact involves absolute judgments obtained independently at different time periods, some before and others after the events.

Both types of assessments are important if we are to understand the psychological costs of disasters. Focused assessments conducted immediately after a traumatic event provide critical prognostic information, identifying those individuals at risk for severe distress and dysfunction (Galea et al., 2002; Norris, Byrne, Diaz, & Kaniasty, 2001). Both the scope and the duration of effects that have emerged from focused assessments have surprised many mental health specialists. In some cases, serious problems have been identified in 60–90% of people exposed to a disaster (Norris et al., 2001; Pine & Cohen, 2002), and these problems may persist for many years (Havenaar et al., 1997; Tyano et al., 1996; Yule et al., 2000).

The ambient domain may provide a broader window on everyday psychological functioning, one with significant value in understanding how people change and in predicting long–term psychological distress that may fall below clinical diagnostic thresholds. Although ambient impact has not been a focus in disaster research, the value of examining such processes is suggested by studies of major life events, both positive and negative. People who experience a serious accident, negotiate a difficult divorce, or even win the lottery apparently return relatively quickly to their preevent levels of subjective well-being (Brickman, Coates, & Janoff-Bulman, 1978; Suh, Diener, & Fujita, 1996). A better understanding of ambient impact promises to inform the critical distinction between serious traumatic reactions and what might be considered normal responses to abnormal events, the former signaling vulnerability to clinical dysfunction or need for intervention, and the latter most likely self-limiting.

Perhaps one reason for the dearth of data on ambient impacts is that they present notable assessment challenges. Such effects are often subtle and elusive and may require measures that are more fine-grained than those provided by standard questionnaires or interview protocols. Documentation of ambient impact also depends on the availability of information about predisaster functioning; given that disasters are by nature sudden and unexpected, such prospective studies pose significant methodological challenges.

The Present Study

Our investigative team has been conducting longitudinal studies of adolescent stress and health for several years. Using a custom electronic diary program installed on handheld computers, adolescents report their moods, contexts, and activities 25-30 times a day for four consecutive days twice each year. The existence of predisaster diaries, along with psychosocial and demographic information collected at the start of the study, affords us a unique opportunity to examine associations between reactions to September 11 and a wealth of data already available on these same adolescents. Because this is an ongoing study, participants had been scheduled before the events of September 11 to repeat the electronic diary phase in the Fall of 2001. Thus we were able to compare dense samples of adolescent moods and states before and after the tragedy.

Specific questions addressed in this study were: (a) Do adolescents distant from the attack sites view themselves as having been affected by the events and as experiencing traumatic symptoms? (b) Do preexisting anxiety or depression levels predict reactions to distant trauma? (c) What are the affective responses of adolescents when asked explicitly about the attacks (focused impact)? and (d) Are there differences in adolescents' everyday emotional functioning assessed before and after but independently of the attacks (ambient impact)? Focused impact was assessed by a self-report questionnaire, similar to those used in other studies, that asked adolescents about their perceptions of and reactions to the events of September 11. Ambient impact was assessed by comparing diary mood ratings following the events of September 11, 2001, with those obtained at the start of the study, between 1 and 3 years earlier.

METHOD

Overview

Since the Fall of 1998, we have enrolled yearly cohorts of high school freshmen (9th-grade students) in a longitudinal investigation of health behaviors and tobacco-use susceptibility called Project MASH (Monitoring Adolescent Stress and Health). The primary component of the ongoing project involves semiannual waves of experience sampling, using electronic diaries, during the four high school years. Before beginning the initial diary wave, each student and a parent attended an orientation session in which all procedures were explained, informed consent was obtained, and teens and parents completed a set of psychosocial questionnaires. After the terrorist attacks of September 11, 2001, all continuing participants were invited to complete a questionnaire about these events. This study examines adolescent perceptions of and reactions to the events of September 11 and compares diary-reported moods before and after these events.

Participants

One hundred seventy-one Project MASH participants (71 males, 100 females) returned completed questionnaires: 44 high school seniors (Fall 1998 cohort),

60 juniors (Fall 1999 cohort), and 67 sophomores (Fall 2000 cohort). These adolescents ranged in age between 14.8 and 18.7 years (M = 16.3, SD = 0.86). The ethnic distribution was 58.5% Caucasian, 17% Asian, 12.9% Latino, 1.2% Black, and 10.5% mixed or other. This was a middle income, well-educated group, with 72% of parents having attended college and 55% having earned a bachelor's or advanced degree.

Measures

September 11, 2001 Reaction Inventory   This 10-page instrument included questions about overall reactions to the attacks, exposure to specific event-related consequences, posttraumatic stress symptoms, and perceptions of how things have changed in the United States. Adolescents were also asked about their moods and physical states (e.g., fatigue) when they first learned of the events of September 11. In November 2001, these surveys were mailed to parents of the 409 adolescents participating in the longitudinal study, and 171 (42%) adolescents returned completed surveys.

For overall reactions, respondents were asked to rate, on a scale from 0 to 100, how much they thought the events of September 11 affected America, other students in their school, themselves, and their future. A separate item asked, "Overall, considering both big ways and little ways that you were touched by the events of September 11, how stressful would you say your life has been since?" The scale ranged from 1 (not stressed) to 10 (extremely stressed).

To measure perceived consequences or exposure, two sets of yes/no items were included, the first focusing on people they knew (e.g., "Do you know anyone who was called up for military service?"), and the second focusing on changes in their own lives (e.g., changes in family rules, activities, or travel plans; see Table I). Each section also included a write-in item asking about any positive changes.

Post-traumatic-stress items (e.g., "Do thoughts about the attacks come back to you even when you do not want them to?"), adapted from Norris (2001) and Vernberg et al. (1996), were rated from 0 (not at all) to 4 (very much). The 14 items were combined into a single posttraumatic Stress Symptom Index (PTSSI). Scores could range from 0 to 56, with higher numbers reflecting greater distress levels. Internal reliability (coefficient alpha) for this scale was .81.

Six-point word scales assessed adolescent moods and states, using the same format that respondents were accustomed to in the electronic diaries. These moods were assessed in three contexts: "right now" (before beginning the survey), "when I first learned about the events," and "thinking about September 11 today." One or more pages of unrelated items separated these three sets of mood ratings. This initial study focused on five major affective states: happiness, anger, sadness, anxiety, and stress.

TABLE I   Perceived Changes As a Result of the Events of September 11

Overall Impact	Girls M (SD) N = 99	Boys M (SD) N = 72	Total M (SD) N = 171
How much do you think the events of September 11th … (0 = not at all–100 = very much, as much as possible)			
affected America	92.01 (14.83)	90.00 (13.92)	91.16 (14.49)
affected you	61.06 (26.38)	48.76 (27.67)★★	55.88 (27.53)
will affect you future	65.80 (24.69)	54.97 (27.16)★★	61.24 (26.23)
affected other students	65.90 (24.91)	55.21 (24.87)★★	61.41 (25.37)
As a result of the events of September 11, do you know anyone who (% yes)			
Lost a job	16.2	13.9	15.2
Had to change to a different job	6.1	8.3	7.0
Job became harder	20.2	18.1	19.4
Was called up for military service	28.3	19.4	24.6
May be called up for military service	41.4	23.6★	34.3
Being a student became harder	21.2	12.5	17.6
Was hurt in the attacks	15.2	15.3	15.2
Positive changes?	36.0	18.2★	28.4
As a result of the events of September 11, changes in your own life (% yes)			
Change in travel plans	31.3	18.1★	25.7
Change in activities or events	37.4	20.8★	30.4
Change in family rules	25.3	11.1★	19.3
Change in use of money	15.2	9.7	13.0
Being a student became harder	0.2	9.7	15.8
Positive changes?	25.3	13.8	20.4

★ $p < .05$. ★★ $p < .01$.

Experience Sampling Using Electronic Diaries

Throughout their high school years, students participated in semiannual experience sampling waves, each extending over four consecutive days, Thursday through Sunday. This interval was selected to ensure dense sampling across a range of naturally occurring events and situations on both school days and weekends and to allow for the inevitable data losses that occur during activities incompatible with diary recording. These waves were scheduled approximately 6 months apart, fall and spring.

Information was collected using a custom diary program that was installed on Palm III handheld computers (3Com, Santa Clara, CA). All other computer functions (e.g., calendar, address book) were locked out. An auditory signal was emitted every 25 ± 10 min during waking hours, yielding approximately 25–30 recording opportunities each day. If a diary entry was not made, up to three reminder signals were emitted at 1-min intervals; the diary then became inaccessible until the next scheduled occurrence.

Students were instructed to do what they normally do during the monitoring days. When they heard the signal, they were to stop what they were doing and complete a diary record, which took about 1 min. They were told to ignore any signal that occurred during an incompatible activity (e.g., bike riding, class test, religious service). Daily start and stop times were programmed individually, according to each student's usual sleep pattern. This electronic diary procedure ensures total confidentiality, even if a palmtop is misplaced or borrowed by curious peers or parents. It also ensures temporal accuracy because participants must complete each diary record soon after the signal and thus cannot delay or clump entries.

Each student was paired with a project coach who met the student at school and kept in touch by phone. On the first day of each 4-day sequence, students were met at school by their coach before classes began. After the diary procedures were reviewed, they were given a toll-free number and encouraged to call at any time with questions or problems. They were also given a project ID card (including the toll-free number) that they could present if questioned by any adult who might wonder why the student is carrying a handheld computer that emits auditory signals. To ensure comfort, comprehension, and compliance, they were revisited at school by their coach on the second day and contacted by phone each evening to review what they had done and discuss any problems. The palmtop computers were collected on Monday morning following the 4-day sequence, and the data were uploaded in the university laboratory.

Several steps were taken to train students to use the electronic diaries. They were introduced to the handheld computers during their orientation session, and they received a "Research Manual" that detailed the procedures and reviewed specific items and decision rules. A brief refresher course was given by the coaches at the beginning of each experience sampling wave, new copies of the manual were distributed, and coaches were on call to answer questions, review progress and procedures, and repair or replace malfunctioning equipment. We have found that adolescents learn the basics quickly and have no difficulties understanding the items, making choices, or entering responses.

To encourage steady compliance after the initial novelty wore off, students were paid $20 for each day they participated, and they earned bonus points for each completed diary record up to an additional $5 per day. Thus for each 4-day sequence they could earn $100. The first day's bonus was paid at the Day 2 check-in and the remaining bonuses when the equipment was returned; the main payment of $80 was mailed. The program provided a password-protected tally of completed diary records so that the coaches could trouble shoot in the field and check compliance. To encourage continuation in the study, the compensation was increased to $120 after 2 years of participation.

The diary contained a fixed sequence of 24 items selected to tap contexts, activities, and moods that are relevant to the daily lives of adolescents. The slate of diary items began by asking "who," "what," and "where," that is, students selected one of several alternatives to indicate their social context (e.g., alone, family, friends); primary activity (e.g., phone, lesson/practice, think/plan); and location (e.g., home, school, mall). They then answered "Yes" or "No" to indicate what they consumed since the last recording (e.g., meal, caffeine, cigarette/tobacco) and whether they were feeling hassled. Ten display screens followed, each containing 6-point word scales that tap specific moods (e.g., anxiety: none, uneasy, tense, worried, pressured, overwhelmed), urges to eat and smoke, and other states (alertness, fatigue). Additional details about the electronic diary procedures and findings appear in Henker, Whalen, Jamner, and Delfino (2002), Whalen, Jamner, Henker, and Delfino (2001), and Whalen, Jamner, Henker, Delfino, and Lozano (2002).

From the diaries, this study focused on the same affective dimensions examined in the surveys: happiness, anger, sadness, anxiety, and stress. For all cohorts, electronic diary data from Wave 1 (beginning of freshman year) were compared to those from Fall 2001, following the September 11 attacks (from mid-September through early December). Thus, these comparisons spanned between 1 and 3 years, depending on the cohort. The decision to use Wave 1 data rather than data from Fall 2000 for all cohorts was based on a number of considerations, including a desire to have all baseline data collected from students comparable in age, grade, and electronic diary experience. Another reason is that Wave 1 diary data were collected in closest temporal proximity to the baseline psychosocial measures. Finally, we felt that including pre-post intervals of 1, 2, and 3 years provided a robust test of the continuity of everyday moods.

Baseline Psychosocial Measures

Prior to the first diary wave, participating adolescents and their parents provided information about the adolescents' internalizing and externalizing problems. Adolescents completed the Youth Self-Report (YSR) and parents completed the Child Behavior Checklist (CBCL), parallel instruments that tap diverse dimensions of child psychopathology and behavior problems (Achenbach, 1991a, 1991b). Ratings of the adolescents' DSM-IV ADHD symptoms were also obtained from both adolescent and parent. The adolescents completed additional questionnaires designed to tap impulsivity (Barratt Impulsivity Scale or BIS; Patton, Stanford, & Barratt, 1995), hostility (Cook-Medley Hostility subscale of the Minnesota Multiphasic Personality Inventory; Cook & Medley, 1954), depression (youth version of the Center for Epidemiological Studies Depression Scale or CES-D; Radloff, 1991), anxiety (Revised Children's Manifest Anxiety Scale or RCMAS; Reynolds & Richmond, 1997), and optimism (Life Orientations Test or LOT; Scheier & Carver, 1985).

Procedures

Because of the possibility that questions about the terrorist attacks could prove upsetting to some adolescents, the survey packets were mailed to parents so that they could decide whether to discuss the study with their teenager. The packet contained two copies of the survey, two stamped self-addressed envelopes, consent forms, and a check for $15. Parents were asked to review the consent form, discuss the study with their teen, and then each could decide whether or not to participate. They were asked to complete the surveys independently, without discussion, and return them separately in the envelopes provided. The $15 was described as a token of appreciation that was for them to keep whether or not they completed the survey. All procedures were approved by the Institutional Review Board of the University of California, Irvine. This paper focuses on responses of the adolescents; comparisons between parent and adolescent reactions will be reported separately.

RESULTS

Sample Comparisons and Adherence

Comparisons between the September 11 survey respondents and the remainder of the sample revealed no differences in age or ethnicity, but there was a somewhat disproportionate number of girls in the survey sample, 58.5%, compared with 49.4% in the full sample (one-sample binomial test, p = .02). On the baseline psychosocial measures, there were no differences in preexisting anxiety (RCMAS) or depression levels (CES-D), but respondents had somewhat lower scores than nonrespondents on externalizing problems, as indicated by parent aggression and delinquency ratings on the CBCL, adolescent self-ratings of delinquency on the YSR and hostility on the Cook-Medley, and parent (but not adolescent) ratings of ADHD using the DSM-IV checklist.

Complete electronic diary data both before and after the attacks were available for 161 of the 171 or 94% of the adolescents who returned completed surveys. Diary adherence rates were quite good. On average, these adolescents completed diaries on 82% of possible occasions, and adherence rates were similar for boys (81%) and girls (83%).

Perceived Effects and Posttraumatic Distress

A substantial number of adolescents experienced changes themselves that they attributed to the events of September 11 and knew people who were affected by major life events such as being called up for military service (Table I). Many reported changes in their own daily lives in domains quite central to adolescents, including family rules (19.3%) and travel plans (25.7%). Of particular interest is that approximately one third of the respondents identified at least one benefit, with 28.4% reporting positive changes in others and a partially overlapping 20.4% reporting positive changes in themselves. These perceived benefits ranged from proximal (self, family, friends) to distal (societal or global). The majority clustered into six categories: greater interpersonal closeness and togetherness, 25.9% (e.g., "I tell my mom I love her now"); increased gratitude and appreciation, 20.4% (e.g., "Value life more and all experiences");

more caring and altruistic acts, 13% (e.g., "Wanting to help out"); growing interest in world events, 11.1% (e.g., "More aware of the goings on around the world"); increased patriotism and national unity, 25.9% (e.g., "America united together for first time in a while"); and enhanced alertness and security, 18.5% (e.g., "Became more aware of my surroundings"; and "Our security has gone up").

When asked simply how much they had been affected overall (using a 0–100 scale, from not at all to very much, as much as possible), these adolescents indicated a moderate impact (M = 55.88) despite being 3,000 miles from the attack sites. They viewed themselves as somewhat less affected than their peers (M = 61.41, t = 3.22, p < .01) and markedly less affected than America (M = 91.16, t = 18.49, p <.001). The difference between self- and peer-ratings may reflect processes similar to those underlying the "optimistic bias" phenomenon that emerges when individuals compare their own risks to those of other people (Weinstein & Klein, 1995; Whalen et al., 1994). For themselves as well as their peers, girls acknowledged a greater impact than boys.

The PTSSI also revealed clear effects. At least 20% of these adolescents responded "somewhat," "quite a bit," or "very much" to questions about having unwanted thoughts about the attacks (20.6%), seeing pictures or hearing sounds in their mind about the attacks (21.1%), and thinking that it might happen again (50.3%). Many adolescents reported not enjoying things as much as before (25.6%), not sleeping well (22.3%), and having more difficulty paying attention (33%). It is important to emphasize that, for most items, the reactions were moderate rather than extreme. When only the two highest scale points were included, endorsement rates were substantially lower, ranging between 5 and 21%. Endorsements of either "quite a bit" or "very much" were highest for "it might happen again" (21.3%), "more difficulty paying attention" (20.6%), and "don't enjoy things as much as before" (13.1%). There were no age differences in the total PTSSI; girls had marginally higher scores than boys (Ms = 13.69 vs. 11.73, t = 1.79, p = .075).

Self-rated anxiety (RCMAS) and depression (CES-D) were both correlated with the PTSSI, rs = .43 and .36, respectively, ps < .001. Given the high rates of cooccurrence of internalizing and externalizing problems, it is not surprising that posttraumatic distress was also predicted by externalizing behaviors such as aggression (YSR, r = .27, p < .001) and impulsivity (BIS, r = .36, p < .001). These associations were found more frequently when adolescents rather than parents provided the assessments. For example, the correlation of the PTSSI with ADHD DSM-IV symptoms was .26, p < .001, for adolescent self-ratings but only .04, ns, for parent ratings using the same scale. Optimism seemed to exert a protective effect, as indicated by an inverse correlation with the PTSSI (r = −.27, p < .001).

To provide a more complete picture of stress reactions, a hierarchical regression analysis was conducted with the PTSSI as the dependent variable. First, age, gender, and elapsed time (time between September 11 and survey

TABLE II Summary of Hierarchical Regression Analysis for Variables Predicting Posttraumatic Stress Symptoms Following the Events of September 11, 2001 (N = 157)

Variable	B	SE B	β
Step 1			
Elapsed time	−1.33	.61	−.17*
Step 2			
Elapsed time	−1.23	.55	−.16*
RCMAS total	.43	.07	.43***
Step 3			
Elapsed time	−1.13	.54	−.15*
RCMAS total	.32	.08	.32***
Anger, Wave 1	−1.44	1.58	−.12
Sadness, Wave 1	.78	1.49	.07
Anxiety, Wave 1	5.20	1.46	.56***
Happiness, Wave 1	−.85	.77	−.08
Stress, Wave 1	−2.49	1.08	−.34*

NOTE: Adjusted R^2 = .26. R^2 = .03 for Step 1 (p < .05). δR^2 = .19 for Step 2 (p < .001). δR^2 = .08 for Step 3 (p < .01). RCMAS = Revised Children's Manifest Anxiety Scale.
* p < .05.
*** p < .001.

completion) were entered as control variables. Next, preexisting trait anxiety (RCMAS) and depression (CES-D) were added as predictors, followed by predisaster (Wave 1) diary mood ratings, and then the interactions of age and gender with CES-D, RCMAS, and PTSSI scores were tested. There were no significant contributions of age, gender, preexisting depression (CES-D), or any of the interactions, so these terms were dropped from the final model. As can be seen in Table II, elapsed time was modestly associated with distress, accounting for 3% of the variance. Preexisting trait anxiety, as indexed by the RCMAS, accounted for another 19% of the variance, and diary anxiety and stress accounted for another 8% of the variance, resulting in an R^2 of .30 and an adjusted R^2 of .26. The incremental contribution of stress was in a direction opposite to that of anxiety, an unexpected finding. Perhaps perceived stress for adolescents contains at least two components, one linked to distressed affect, and hence correlated with anxiety, and another reflecting a busy lifestyle. In a preliminary model, externalizing scores (aggression, delinquency, and ADHD) were added but made no incremental contribution. In summary, self-reports of September 11-related traumatic distress were predicted by preexisting anxiety levels as measured by a traditional global questionnaire (RCMAS) and by aggregated contemporaneous diary reports of anxious feelings, with each approach making an independent contribution.

Focused Versus Ambient Impact on Moods

When asked explicitly about the events of September 11, these adolescents reported markedly elevated levels of negative affect. Mean ratings of anger, anxiety, and sadness when first learning about the events of September 11 were 2.58, 2.32, and 2.78, respectively. For comparison purposes, means for these three moods during pre–September 11 experience sampling waves were .62, .75, and .45, respectively, on these 0–5 scales.

When adolescents did not have their attention drawn to the attacks, however, there was no evidence of elevated levels of everyday negative affect after the attacks. For neither girls nor boys did the mean levels of anger, anxiety, stress, sadness, or happiness differ in the electronic diaries between the initial wave of experience sampling and the postattack Fall 2001 wave (see Fig. 1).

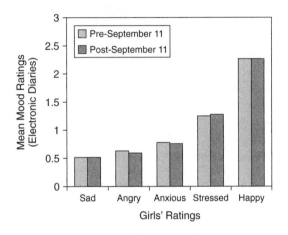

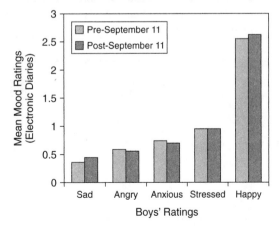

FIGURE 1   Assessing ambient impact: Comparisons of diary-recorded moods, by gender, between experience sampling waves that occurred before and after September 11, 2001.

Negative mood levels were not significantly higher after September 11 for any cohort, that is, for comparisons that spanned 1, 2, or 3 years. Gender differences in stress and happiness emerged in both experience sampling waves: In comparison with boys, girls reported higher levels of stress and lower levels of happiness. In summary, when not asked explicitly about the attacks, adolescents reported mood levels following the attacks that were comparable to those recorded 1–3 years earlier. We also examined the variability of moods and found no significant pre-post differences.

As a further test of the effects of September 11 on everyday anxiety levels, a regression analysis was conducted with diary anxiety level during Fall 2001 as the dependent variable. Age and gender were entered at Step 1 as control variables, followed by trait anxiety and depression (Step 2), then the PTSSI (Step 3), preexisting diary anxiety levels (Step 4), and finally the interaction terms (Step 5). Once again, there were no significant effects of age, gender, or CES-D, nor did any of the interactions reach significance, so these variables were removed from the final model. As can be seen in Table III, the diary measure of pre-September 11 (Wave 1) anxiety was the primary predictor of postdisaster anxiety levels, yielding an adjusted R^2 of .49. Although trait anxiety (RCMAS) was associated with post-September 11 diary anxiety, it made no incremental contribution over pre-September 11 diary anxiety. Posttraumatic distress made no contribution at any stage of analysis.

To provide a more detailed view of the affective terrain, 4 (mood rating context) x 2 (gender) analyses of variance were used to compare self-ratings in the Fall 2001 diaries with the three ratings from the September 11 Reaction Inventory: current feelings, feelings when first learning of the attacks, and feelings now when thinking back to the attacks. All mood context main effects

TABLE III Summary of Hierarchical Regression Analysis for Variables Predicting Post-September 11 Diary Anxiety (N = 150)

Variable	B	SE B	β
Step 1			
RCMAS total	.04	.01	.35***
Step 2			
RCMAS total	.03	.01	.31***
Posttraumatic stress symptoms	.01	.01	.11
Step 3			
RCMAS total	.004	.01	.04
Posttraumatic stress symptoms	−.007	.01	−.07
Diary anxiety at Wave 1	.67	.06	.71***

NOTE: Adjusted R^2 = .49. R^2 = .12 for Step 1 (p = .001). δR^2 = .01 for Step 2 (ns). δR^2 = .37 for Step 3 (p < .001). RCMAS = Revised Children's Manifest Anxiety Scale.
*** p < .001.

were significant, and each profile revealed the expected rank order. The "thinking back" ratings fell midway between ratings of current moods and remembered moods (when first learning of the attacks). There were no differences between current mood ratings on the survey and average mood ratings obtained from the Fall 2001 electronic diaries. Overall, girls compared with boys reported higher levels of sadness and stress, marginally higher levels of anxiety (p = .065), and lower levels of happiness but, interestingly, comparable levels of anger. For sadness, the mood rating Context x Gender interaction was also significant, reflecting the emergence of larger gender differences in questionnaire than in electronic diary ratings.

DISCUSSION

Four primary findings emerged from this study. First, adolescents distant from the disaster sites did indeed view themselves as having been affected significantly by the events: For example, 30% perceived changes in everyday life activities and many also reported putative PTSD symptoms. Second, these distress indicators were predicted by preexisting anxiety levels and not by age, gender, or externalizing problems. Third, elevated levels of negative affect emerged when adolescents were asked how they reacted to the events (focused impact) but not when their ongoing, momentary mood reports before and after the events were compared (ambient impact). In other words, elevated negative affect was reported when the salience of the events was underscored. When these adolescents reported on contemporary feelings without having their attention directed toward September 11, mood levels were comparable to those recorded 1-3 years before the terror attacks. Fourth, a traditional trait measure (RCMAS) and aggregated, contemporaneous state measures (electronic diary reports) of anxiety each made independent contributions to the prediction of distress following the attacks.

Reactions to Distant Traumas

The exposure items included in this survey were relatively mild in the context of the severe losses, injuries, and disruptions sustained by many people who lived closer to the attack sites. In some instances, the exposure items can be characterized as reflecting changes rather than traumatic events. Alterations in everyday routines and family life can have a significant impact during adolescence, however, especially for those already vulnerable because of preexisting problems or other environmental stressors. Recent studies indicate that even partial or subthreshold PTSD symptoms can be associated with impaired functioning, and that trauma reactions are more accurately construed as dimensional than as categorical, with PTSD located at the extreme end of a stress-response continuum (Ruscio, Ruscio, & Keane, 2002; Shear, 2002). Although meaningful numbers of this community sample of adolescents reported stress reactions, it is unlikely that these reactions were severe or enduring enough to suggest clinical intervention. They may, however, indicate the merits of providing supportive services for adolescents exposed to major tragedies, even when exposure is based more on media reports than personal experiences.

Especially noteworthy is the finding that a third of these adolescents acknowledged salutary effects on themselves or others at the same time they were itemizing the negative consequences. Some perceived greater interpersonal closeness and caring, whereas others focused on national and global benefits. This process of identifying "silver linings," which has also emerged in studies of adults who experience personal traumas, may reflect an adaptive coping response. People often manage their distress and regulate their emotions by reframing and finding new meaning in major illnesses, injuries, or losses (Tedeschi & Calhoun, 1995). The fact that these adolescents estimated the impact on America as far greater than the impact on themselves may reflect what has been called optimistic bias as well as a coping style involving self-reassurance through social comparison.

Strengths and Limitations

The availability of predisaster measures of psycho-social functioning as well as high-density electronic diary mood ratings is a notable strength of this study. This strength must be balanced, however, against a number of limitations. This was not a representative sample of adolescents residing in southern California, but rather a self-selected subgroup from an ongoing longitudinal study that involves semiannual assessments. Adolescents with high levels of personal or family problems were unlikely to enroll or, once enrolled, to continue in the larger study, and those from the larger sample who showed the highest levels of externalizing problems were underrepresented in this study. Whether adolescents with serious externalizing problems reacted in distinctive ways to the events of September 11 remains an open question.

The Promise of Electronic Diaries in Research and Practice

These findings also indicate the value of electronic diary data. The expected association emerged between September 11-related distress and preexisting anxiety levels, as indexed by a frequently used anxiety self-report questionnaire, the RCMAS. The aggregated diary samples were not redundant with this questionnaire but rather provided incremental predictive power. As described and demonstrated in previous studies (e.g., Henker et al., 2002; Whalen et al., 2002), electronic diary approaches have a number of distinct advantages, including precision, contemporaneousness, and high-density sampling. They are not subject to the distortions introduced either by global or by retrospective questions, and they encourage candor by ensuring confidentiality. With continuing technological advances, software developments, and cost reductions, these methodologies should become more accessible and useful to practitioners as well as researchers for the assessment of symptoms-in-context and treatment outcomes in natural environments.

Conclusion

The reports of distinct effects of the September 11 events by adolescents residing 3,000 miles from Ground Zero suggest the value of programs and interventions designed not only to treat clinical disorders but also to help healthy adolescents cope with unprecedented horrors. In fact, the continuing consequences of the attacks of September 11 provide critical "teaching moments," ongoing opportunities to enhance affect regulation and coping skills in adolescents that may serve a long-term protective function as these young people mature and experience future stressors. Importantly, there was no evidence that the mood and behavior patterns reported by these adolescents index psychopathology. Rather, their negative reactions may be self-limiting. Although explicit questioning may increase the salience of stressful memories, there may be no detectable changes in daily functioning when attention is not directed to the traumatic events. Striking the optimal balance between minimizing and exacerbating adolescents' normal reactions to abnormal events is a major challenge for researchers and clinicians alike.

REFERENCES

Achenbach, T.M. (1991a). *Manual for the Child Behavior Checklist/4-18 and 1991 profile.* Burlington: University of Vermont, Department of Psychiatry.

Achenbach, T.M. (1991b). *Manual for the Youth Self-Report and 1991 profile.* Burlington: University of Vermont, Department of Psychiatry.

Asarnow, J., Glynn, S., Pynoos, R. S., Nahum, J., Guthrie, D., Cantwell, D. P., et al. (1999). When the earth stops shaking: Earthquake sequelae among children diagnosed for pre-earthquake psychopathology. *Journal of the American Academy of Child & Adolescent Psychiatry, 38,* 1016–1023.

Brickman, P., Coates, D., & Janoff-Bulman, R. (1978). Lottery winners and accident victims: Is happiness relative? *Journal of Personality and Social Psychology, 36,* 917–927.

Centers for Disease Control and Prevention. (2002). Psychological and emotional effects of the September 11 attacks on the World Trade Center—Connecticut, New Jersey, and New York, 2001. *Morbidity and Mortality Weekly Report, 51,* 784–786.

Cook, W. W., & Medley, D. M. (1954). Proposed hostility and pharisaic-virtue scales for the MMPI. *Journal of Applied Psychology, 39,* 414–418.

Galea, S., Ahern, J., Resnick, H., Kilpatrick, D., Bucuvalas, M., Gold, J., et al. (2002). Psychological sequelae of the September 11 terrorist attacks in New York City. *New England Journal of Medicine, 346,* 982–987.

Halpern-Felsher, B.L., & Millstein, S. G. (2002). The effects of terrorism on teens' perceptions of dying: The new world is riskier than ever. *Journal of Adolescent Health, 30,* 308–311.

Havenaar, J. M., Rumyantzeva, G. M., van den Brink, W., Poelijoe, N. W., van den Bout, J., van Engeland, H., et al. (1997). Long-term mental health effects of the Chernobyl disaster: An epidemiologic survey in two former Soviet regions. *American Journal of Psychiatry, 154,* 1605–1607.

Henker, B., Whalen, C. K., Jamner, L. D., & Delfino, R. J. (2002). Anxiety, affect, and activity in teenagers: Monitoring daily life with electronic diaries. *Journal of the American Academy of Child & Adolescent Psychiatry, 41,* 660–670.

Katz, C. L., Pellegrino, L., Pandya, A., Ng, A., & DeLisi, L. E. (2002). Research on psychiatric outcomes and interventions subsequent to disasters: A review of the literature. *Psychiatry Research, 110,* 201–217.

La Greca, A. M., Silverman, W. K., & Wasserstein, S. B. (1998). Children's predisaster functioning as a predictor of posttraumatic stress following Hurricane Andrew. *Journal of Consulting and Clinical Psychology, 66,* 883–892.

Norris, F. H. (2001). *Measuring exposure to the events of September 11, 2001: Pretest results and stress/loss norms obtained from a minimally exposed but diverse sample of college students.* Retrieved November 5, 2001, from http://obssr.od.nih.gov/Activities/911/attack.htm

Norris, F. H., Byrne, C. M., Diaz, E., & Kaniasty, K. (2001). *50,000 disaster victims speak: An empirical review of the empirical literature, 1981–2001.* Report prepared for The National Center for PTSD and The Center for Mental Health Services (SAMHSA). Retrieved November 5, 2001, from http://obssr.od.nih.gov/Activities/911/disaster-impact.pdf

Patton, J. H., Stanford, M. S., & Barratt, E. S. (1995). Factor structure of the Barratt Impulsiveness Scale. *Journal of Clinical Psychology, 51,* 768–774.

Pfefferbaum, B. (1997). Posttraumatic stress disorder in children: A review of the past 10 years. *Journal of the American Academy of Child & Adolescent Psychiatry, 36,* 1503–1511.

Pine, D. S., & Cohen, J. A. (2002). Trauma in children and adolescents: Risk and treatment of psychiatric sequelae. *Biological Psychiatry, 51,* 519–531.

Pynoos, R. S., Nader, K., Frederick, C., Gonda, L., & Stuber, M. (1987). Grief reactions in school-age children following a sniper attack at school. *Israeli Journal of Psychiatry, 24,* 53–63.

Radloff, L. S. (1991). The use of the Center for Epidemiologic Studies Depression Scale in adolescents and young adults. *Journal of Youth and Adolescence, 20,* 149–166.

Reynolds, C. R., & Richmond, B. O. (1997). What I think and feel: A revised measure of children's manifest anxiety. *Journal of Abnormal Child Psychology, 25,* 15–20.

Ruscio, A. M., Ruscio, J., & Keane, T. M. (2002). The latent structure of posttraumatic stress disorder: A taxometric investigation of reactions to extreme stress. *Journal of Abnormal Psychology, 111,* 290–301.

Scheier, M. F., & Carver, C. S. (1985). Optimism, coping, and health: Assessment and implications of generalized outcome expectancies. *Health Psychology, 4,* 219–247.

Schuster, M. A., Stein, B. D., Jaycox, L. H., Collins, R. L., Marshall, G. N., Elliott, M. N., et al. (2001). A national survey of stress reactions after the September 11, 2001, terrorist attacks. *New England Journal of Medicine, 345,* 1507–1512.

Shear, M. K. (2002). Building a model of posttraumatic stress disorder. *American Journal of Psychiatry, 159,* 1631–1633.

Silver, R. C., Holman, E. A., McIntosh, D. N., Poulin, M., & Gil-Rivas, V. (2002). Nationwide longitudinal study of psychological responses to September 11, *JAMA, 288,* 1235–1244.

Suh, E., Diener, E., & Fujita, F. (1996). Events and subjective well-being: Only recent events matter. *Journal of Personality and Social Psychology, 70,* 1091–1102.

Tedeschi, R. G., & Calhoun, L. G. (1995). *Trauma and transformation: Growing in the aftermath of suffering,* Thousand Oaks, CA: Sage.

Terr, L. C., Bloch, D. A., Michel, B. A., Shi, H., Reinhardt, J. A., & Metayer, S. (1997). Children's thinking in the wake of Challenger. *American Journal of Psychiatry, 154,* 744–751.

Terr, L. C., Bloch, D. A., Michel, B. A., Shi, H., Reinhardt, J. A., & Metayer, S. (1999). Children's symptoms in the wake of Challenger: A field study of distant-traumatic effects and an outline of related conditions. *American Journal of Psychiatry, 156,* 1536–1544.

Tyano, S., Iancu, I., Solomon, Z., Sever, J., Goldstein, I., Touviana, Y., et al. (1996). Seven-year follow-up of child survivors of a bus-train collision. *Journal of the American Academy of Child & Adolescent Psychiatry, 35,* 365–373.

Vernberg, E. M., La Greca, A. M., Silverman, W. K., & Prinstein, M. J. (1996). Prediction of posttraumatic stress symptoms in children after Hurricane Andrew. *Journal of Abnormal Psychology, 105,* 237–248.

Weinstein, N. D., & Klein, W. M. (1995). Resistance of personal risk perceptions to debiasing interventions. *Health Psychology, 14,* 132–140.

Whalen, C. K., Henker, B., O'Neil, R., Hollingshead, J., Holman, A., & Moore, B. (1994). Optimism in children's judgments of health and environmental risks. *Health Psychology, 13,* 319–325.

Whalen, C. K., Jamner, L. D., Henker, B., & Delfino, R. J. (2001). Smoking and moods in adolescents with depressive and aggressive dispositions: Evidence from surveys and electronic diaries. Health Psychology, 20, 99–111.

Whalen, C. K., Jamner, L. D., Henker, B., Delfino, R. J., & Lozano, J. M. (2002). The ADHD spectrum and everyday life: Experience sampling of adolescent moods, activities, smoking, and drinking. Child Development, 73, 209–227.

Yule, W., Bolton, D., Udwin, O., Boyle, S., O'Ryan, D., & Nurrish, J. (2000). The long-term psychological effects of a disaster experienced in adolescence: I. The incidence and course of PTSD. Journal of Child Psychology and Psychiatry, 41, 503–511.

Yule, W., Perrin, S., & Smith, P. (2001). Traumatic events and post-traumatic stress disorder. In W. K. Silverman & P. D. A. Treffers (Eds.), Anxiety disorders in children and adolescents: Research, assessment and intervention (pp. 212–234). New York: Cambridge University Press.

DISCUSSION QUESTIONS

1. Explain the difference between focused and ambient impact. Why is it important to study the ambient impact of events.

2. What was the purpose of this study? What were the authors trying to find out?

3. What were some of the post-traumatic stress symptoms that adolescents reported having?

4. What were some of the positive outcomes from the attacks that adolescents reported?

5. What did the authors find? Did the September 11th attacks have both a focused and ambient impact? Why do the authors think they found this pattern of results?

6

Gender Differences in Pain Perception: The Mediating Role of Self-Efficacy Beliefs

Todd Jackson, Tony Iezzi, Jennifer Gunderson,
Takeo Nagasaka, and April Fritch

ABSTRACT

The purpose of this study was to assess the extent to which the gender differences in response to the cold pressor test (CPT) are mediated by self-efficacy beliefs. One hundred twelve college undergraduates (69 women and 43 men) engaged in CPT and completed self-report measures of demographic information, physical self-efficacy (i.e., expectations about one's overall physical capabilities), and task-specific self-efficacy (i.e., beliefs about one's ability to cope successfully with the upcoming CPT). In addition, participants provided subjective ratings of pain intensity every 30 s during CPT and were evaluated for tolerance during CPT (up to 4 mm). Consistent with past research, men reported lower average subjective ratings of pain intensity and showed higher tolerance for CPT. Path analyses indicated that associations between gender and pain perception were fully mediated by self-efficacy beliefs. Men reported greater physical self-efficacy and task-specific self-efficacy than women did. In turn, higher task-specific self-efficacy ratings predicted increases in tolerance for pain and lower ratings of average

Sex Roles: A Journal of Research, Dec 2002 p561(8).
"Gender Differences in Pain Perception: The Mediating Role of Self-Efficacy Beliefs" by Todd Jackson, Tony Iezzi, Jennifer Gunderson, Takeo Nagasaka, and April Fritch.© 2002 Plenum Publishing Corporation

pain intensity. Findings indicate that self-efficacy beliefs are one factor that accounts for gender differences in responses to painful stimulation. Future researchers should evaluate conditions under which heightened self-efficacy may be beneficial and harmful, and they should employ experimental designs that incorporate opportunities for use of both communal-interpersonal and individualistic coping strategies in light of possible gender differences in preferred approaches to coping with pain.

INTRODUCTION

An expanding literature indicates that gender is an important influence on experiences of pain. Authors who have reviewed studies of clinical and laboratory pain (e.g., Fillingim, 2000; Riley, Robinson, Wise, Myers, & Fillingim, 1998; Robinson, Riley, & Myers, 2000; Rollman, Lautenbacher, & Jones, 2000; Unruh, 1996) have generally concluded that women and men differ in their perceptions and experiences of pain. For example, Unruh (1996) reviewed research on clinical pain and found that women were more likely than men to experience recurrent pain, as well as frequent, severe, and longer-lasting pain. Women also tended to experience more pain-related disability and to receive unwarranted psychogenic attributions for pain by health professionals from whom they sought treatment. Reviewers e.g., Rollman et al., 2000) have also concluded that women typically report greater sensitivity to and less tolerance for experimentally induced noxious stimulation than men do. Despite these generalizations, some studies of clinical pain (e.g., Faull & Nichol, 1986; Lester, Lefebre, & Keefe, 1994) and experimental pain (e.g., Lautenbacher, Moeltner, & Strian, 1991; Sullivan, Bishop, & Pivik, 1995; Sullivan, Rouse, Bishop, & Johnston, 1997) have not demonstrated gender differences in perception of pain. Methodological considerations regarding sample size (e.g., Sullivan et al., 1995), gender of experimenter (e.g., Levine & de Simone, 1991), and kind of noxious stimulation used (e.g., Rollman et al., 2000) may partially explain inconsistencies. However, discrepant findings also suggest that gender per se may be less important than factors related to gender in explaining links between gender and pain.

Notwithstanding the large body of work on gender differences in pain perception, comparably less is known about specific mechanisms that underlie gender differences in responsiveness to pain. Self-efficacy is one plausible factor that may mediate the relation between gender and pain, in light of its associations with both gender and pain perception. Bandura (1997) defined self-efficacy as an expectation that one can successfully perform behaviors necessary to produce a successful outcome. Typically, heightened self-efficacy is associated with the decision to engage in a behavior, increased effort toward reaching goals, and greater perseverance in the face of obstacles.

Parent and peer group expectations that males be physically strong and media portrayals of men's physical strength, endurance, and athleticism may foster expectations of physical competence among men (Bandura, 1997). These differential patterns of socialization may contribute to the gender gap in physical self-efficacy and performance of physical tasks. Several studies support these ideas. For example, Wittig, Duncan, and Schurr (1987) found that female college students reported a lower mean level of physical self-efficacy than did male students. They also observed an association between physical self-efficacy and endorsements of masculine gender role for both women and men, which suggests that, through socialization, masculinity becomes associated with physical activity. Research on older adults (e.g., Godin & Shephard, 1985) has also shown that women generally tend to report lower physical self-efficacy than do men. Despite its link with gender, the impact of physical self-efficacy on pain perception has not been investigated. Nonetheless, it is reasonable to speculate that people who perceive themselves to be more physically capable should perform better on physically challenging tasks that demand strength and endurance in the face of pain than those who view themselves as less physically capable.

Although there is considerable research on gender differences in self-efficacy related to areas such as occupational aspirations and pursuits, the development of quantitative skills, and risk for depression (e.g., Bandura, 1997; Bussey & Bandura, 1999), there has been surprisingly little research on the association between gender and self-efficacy beliefs related to pain perception. In a qualitative study, Bendelow (1993) found that people recalled that they had learned at a very young age how to respond to pain. In particular, during childhood, men recalled being actively discouraged from expressing their emotions and feeling obligated to display stoicism in response to pain. In contrast, women may have a greater tendency to engage in an interpersonal or a communal approach to coping (e.g., Sullivan, Tripp, & Santor, 2000). In this context, expressions of distress or pain may function to signal a need for interpersonal support. Consequently, self-efficacy for intra-personal ways of coping with pain may be relatively lower among women because it is less relevant to their preferred ways of coping. To date, only one study has directly evaluated gender differences in efficacy for coping with pain. Weisenberg, Tepper, and Schwarzwald (1995) compared 40 healthy men with 40 healthy women on performance during the cold pressor test (CPT). They found that men exhibited higher self-efficacy for pain control than women did. Unfortunately, the authors did not examine whether gender differences in cold pressor tolerance persisted after controlling for self-efficacy beliefs related to pain control.

Other indirect evidence for self-efficacy as a potential mediator of gender differences in pain perception is suggested by recent studies (Keefe et al., 2000; Sullivan et al., 2000) that have shown that catastrophizing may explain gender differences in pain. Logically, individuals who view pain as terrible and overwhelming should also report reduced self-efficacy in its management. Self-efficacy and catastrophizing seem to be related and may even reflect aspects of a higher order construct such as secondary appraisal (Lazarus, 1999), but they are distinct in at least two ways. First, although increased catastrophizing is likely related to reduced self-efficacy, decreased self-efficacy regarding an event does not necessarily mean one will catastrophize or feel overwhelmed by it. Second, in laboratory research on pain perception, initial assessments of self-efficacy are typically conducted before participants are exposed to noxious stimulation, whereas initial assessments of catastrophizing are undertaken during or after exposure to noxious stimulation. Thus, although research on catastrophizing suggests that self-efficacy might mediate the relation between gender and pain perception, direct assessment of self-efficacy is warranted on both conceptual and methodological grounds.

Although there are few data available on gender differences in pain-related efficacy beliefs, the contention that pain sufferers with high self-efficacy are more likely to activate coping responses, persist in coping with pain, and reduce distressing anticipations that elicit arousal (Bandura, O'Leary, Taylor, Gauthier, & Gossard, 1987) has been supported. For example, among college students, heightened self-efficacy for coping with pain predicts longer tolerance times for cold pressor pain (e.g., Baker & Kirsh, 1991; Dolce, Doleys, Raczynski, & Lassie, 1986; Williams & Kinney, 1991). Self-efficacy for the ability to regulate pain intensity also predicts threshold and tolerance for pressure pain (Stevens, Ohlwein, & Catanzaro, 2000). Self-efficacy expectations can even determine responses to noxious stimulation. For example, Litt (1988) manipulated self-efficacy expectancies for pain tolerance by giving false feedback on participants' capacity for tolerance that was independent of their actual tolerance. Tolerance for subsequent pain covaried with self-efficacy and differed from the tolerance and self-efficacy ratings of a control group not given false feedback. Increasing self-efficacy expectancies related to the ability to control pain through biofeedback has also been found to predict reductions in intensity of tension headache (Holroyd et al., 1984).

The evidence cited previously suggests that self-efficacy may contribute to gender differences in pain perception, although this proposition has not been examined directly. The current study was designed to test the hypothesis that gender differences in pain perception are mediated by self-efficacy beliefs. It was hypothesized that men would report higher levels of physical self-efficacy and task-specific self-efficacy (i.e., beliefs about ability to cope with CPT) than women would. In turn, it was expected that the association between gender and pain perception would be mediated by self-efficacy expectations. Specifically, we expected that associations between (1) gender and pain tolerance and (2) gender and pain intensity would vanish after controlling for the impact of physical and task-specific self-efficacy.

METHOD

Participants

The sample was composed of 69 women and 43 men between 17 and 53 years of age (M 22.34, SD 6.25). Most participants were single (90.3%) and White (91.2%). There was no age difference between women (M = 22.88,

SD = 7.02) and men (M 21.48, SD = 4.73), t = 1.3l, p < .44, nor did the women (M = 13.69, SD 3.32) and men (M = 13.50, SD = 2.69) differ in their total years of education, t = 0.10, p < .90.

Measures

Physical Self-Efficacy Scale. (PSE; Ryckman, Robbins, Thornton, & Cantrell, 1982) The PSE is a 22-item measure of perceived physical self-efficacy with underlying dimensions that are related to perceived physical ability (e.g., "My physique is rather strong") and physical self-presentation confidence (e.g., "I am sometimes envious of people who are better looking than me"). Each item was rated on a 6-point scale of agreement/disagreement; higher scores reflected greater physical self-efficacy. The PSE had an alpha coefficient of .83 in this study. Past researchers have found the measure to have a satisfactory 6-week test-retest reliability, r = .85, and associations with participation in athletics and use of physical skills (Ryckman et al., 1982).

Task-Specific Self-Efficacy. A four-item Self-Efficacy Scale (SES) was created by the authors to examine expectations about coping with CPT. The items, rated on a 5-point scale ranging from Not at All to Very Much, assessed participants' degree of certainty that they would be able to control the pain associated with CPT, cope well during CPT, perform the experimental task successfully, and not be able to manage the pain related to CPT (reverse-scored). Alpha coefficients for these four items were .81 in this study and .85 in a recent study (Jackson et al., 2002).

Coping. After completion of the experimental task, participants were asked, "What did you think and do to cope with the cold pressor test?" Coping responses reported were coded on the basis of their consistency with item content of the Coping Strategies Questionnaire (Rosenstiel & Keefe, 1983) subscales—Diverting Attention (e.g., "thought about what I have to do today," "tried to think about other things"), Coping Self Statements (e.g., "felt I could handle this," "no matter how much it hurt, I was going to finish"), Catastrophizing (e.g., "felt like I couldn't stand it anymore"), Pain Behavior/Pain Focus (e.g., "tried moving my fingers," "thought about how much it hurt"), Ignoring Pain Sensations (e.g., "didn't think about it," "just tried to just ignore the pain"), and Reinterpreting Pain Sensations (e.g., "it felt like numbness not pain," "used the pain to remember good times I had as a child during the winter when my hands and feet were cold"). Response content that did not clearly fit any of these categories was classified as Miscellaneous. The overall rate of agreement between two raters who coded either presence or absence of each coping strategy was 94.7%; the remaining discrepancies were discussed with the first author until a consensus was reached.

Pain Tolerance and Pain Intensity. Pain tolerance, operationalized as the total time a participant kept his or her hand in the ice water, was measured with a stopwatch and rounded off to the nearest second. Pain intensity was assessed by calculating the average Subjective Units of Distress Scale

(SUDS) rating from separate SUDS ratings given at each 30-s interval, up to 4 min.

Procedure

Volunteers were recruited from undergraduate psychology classes at the University of Wisconsin–Superior and received course credit for participation. Exclusion criteria included an existing pain condition, a circulatory disorder, high blood pressure, a heart condition, Raynaud's disease, a previous serious cold injury, and/or problems with blood clotting.

Standardized procedures and instructions were used in the experiment. Upon arriving for the experimental session, each participant read and signed the informed consent form. Aside from the task-specific self-efficacy items, which were completed immediately before CPT, other self-report measures were administered in a counterbalanced fashion either before or after CPT. Prior to CPT, participants were instructed by one of four experimenters (two women and two men) how to provide a verbal SUDS rating of pain intensity, using a 0–10-point scale with 0 being no pain at all and 10 being the worst pain you have ever experienced. Next, they were instructed to immerse their nondominant hands fully up to their wrists in a container of room temperature water for 10–15 s to stabilize skin temperature. Finally, volunteers immersed the same hands in a container of ice water maintained at 0–3° C as long as they could, up to a maximum of 4 min. A digital thermometer was used to ensure that water temperature was the same across groups. An experimenter stood directly behind each participant during CPT and requested a verbal SUDS rating of discomfort every 30 s. No other verbal interactions were permitted during this task.

RESULTS

A preliminary analysis indicated that women and men did not differ in their frequency of being tested by a female or male experimenter, $\chi^2(1) = 2.11$, $p < .22$. Moreover, temperature of ice water at termination of CPT did not differ for women and men, $t = 0.47$, $p < $ ns. Subsequently, a multivariate analysis of variance (MANOVA) revealed a significant effect for gender on the research measures, $F(4, 105) = 6.30$, $p < .001$. Table I provides descriptive statistics for women and men on the individual measures. As illustrated there, women reported lower levels of physical and task specific self-efficacy, heightened pain sensitivity, and reduced pain tolerance. Intercorrelations between gender, measures of self-efficacy, average pain intensity, and pain tolerance were all statistically significant (see Table II). Therefore, gender and both measures of self-efficacy beliefs were included as predictors in separate path models for (1) pain tolerance and (2) pain intensity.

TABLE I   Descriptive Statistics and Univariate F Values for Research Measures (N = 112)

Variable	Women		Men	
	Mean	SD	Mean	SD
Physical self-efficacy	84.34	14.11	95.86	10.36
Task-specific self-efficacy	14.13	2.83	15.58	2.46
Average pain intensity	6.27	1.84	5.40	1.75
Total pain tolerance (in seconds)	174.86	87.18	208.12	61.92

Variable	F	p
Physical self-efficacy	21.36	.0001
Task-specific self-efficacy	7.61	.007
Average pain intensity	6.11	.02
Total pain tolerance (in seconds)	4.76	.03

TABLE II   Intercorrelations Between Measures Included in Path Analyses (N = 112)

Variable	1	2	3	4	5
1. Gender	—				
2. Physical self-efficacy	.40***	—			
3. Task-specific self-efficacy	.26**	.40***	—		
4. Total pain tolerance	.21*	.24**	.23**	—	
5. Average pain intensity	−.23*	−.25**	−.24**	−.53***	—

* p < .05.
** p < .01.
*** p < .001.

On the basis of Darlington's recommendations (Darlington, 1990), hierarchical multiple regression analyses were conducted to determine path coefficients (i.e., standardized regression coefficients) between measures in each path model. In the first regression equation, gender was regressed on physical self-efficacy. In the second equation, self-efficacy for CPT was the criterion variable predicted by physical self-efficacy in the first step and gender in the second step of the equation. In the final regression equation, pain tolerance was the criterion variable, predicted by task-specific self-efficacy in Step 1, physical self efficacy in Step 2, and gender in Step 3 of the model. For each equation, t tests based on standardized regression coefficients determined the statistical significance of path coefficients.

Gender and physical self-efficacy had a significant direct association with one another, t = 4.56, p < .0001. Also consistent with predictions, after controlling for gender, physical self-efficacy was related to task-specific self-efficacy,

$t = 2.67$, $p < .009$. Finally, consistent with predictions, high levels of task-specific self-efficacy were associated with increased tolerance for pain, $t = 2.67$, $p < .009$, although neither gender, $t = 1.05$, $p <$ ns, nor physical self-efficacy, $t = 1.65$, $p < .10$, had significant associations with pain tolerance times. Similarly, the association between gender and average pain intensity was also mediated by self-efficacy beliefs; average pain intensity had a negative relation with task-specific self-efficacy, $t = -2.50$, $p < .01$, but not gender, $t = -1.37$, $p <$ ns, or physical self-efficacy, $t = -1.75$, $p < .08$.

Supplementary analyses of post-CPT interview data on coping strategies indicated that 70.5% of the participants reported having diverted attention and 36.6% reported having ignored pain sensations; no other strategy was endorsed by more than 25% of respondents, although 63.7% of the participants used more than one coping strategy during CPT. There were two gender differences in coping strategies endorsed; 81.4% of men and 63.8% of women reported having diverted attention, $\chi^2(1) = 3.96$, $p < .05$, and 26.1% of women and 7.0% of men reported having reinterpreted pain sensations, $\chi^2(1) = 6.35$, $p < .01$. Only two measures of coping were associated with pain perception: use of diverting attention was correlated with increased pain tolerance, $r = .30$, $p < .001$, and focusing on pain was related to increased pain intensity, $r = .30$, $p < .001$.

DISCUSSION

Previous researchers have found relatively consistent gender differences in the perception of pain (e.g., Riley et al., 1998; Unruh, 1996) and in self-efficacy expectations (e.g., Weisenberg et al., 1995; Wittig et al., 1987). However, this is the first study, to our knowledge, to indicate that gender differences in pain perception may be partially a function of self-efficacy beliefs. Two path analyses showed that women reported lower levels of overall physical self-efficacy and self-efficacy in coping with CPT. In turn, reduced self-efficacy beliefs predicted both reduced tolerance for cold pressor pain and increased pain intensity during CPT. After controlling for self-efficacy beliefs, gender was no longer related to either pain tolerance or pain intensity. Together, differences in perceptions of physical capabilities and expectations specifically related to coping with pain accounted for gender differences in sensitivity to and tolerance for cold pressor pain.

Perhaps socialization practices that encourage stoicism and physical robustness among men (e.g., Bendelow, 1993) and the expression of distress among women in order to elicit others' support (e.g., Lyons & Sullivan, 1998; Sullivan et al., 2000) contribute to gender differences in self-efficacy and pain perception. Regardless of how they arise, such gender differences can have both positive and negative effects. On the one hand, keeping in mind that pain is a warning signal for possible tissue damage, women's greater sensitivity to pain can help to protect them from harmful effects of acute injury or disease

(Gijsbers & Niven, 1995). As Unruh (1996) asserted, women learn to attend to pain sooner than men, in part, because injuries or diseases that give rise to pain often result in greater interference in women's abilities to meet occupational, parenting, and household responsibilities. In the same context, extremely high levels of efficacy regarding physical competence and ability to cope with pain may increase risk of harm. For example, when chest and arm pain are indicative of heart attack, the tendency to "grin and bear it" may lead to delays in seeking medical attention that is clearly warranted.

In contrast, low levels of self-efficacy may contribute to increases in suffering in other contexts. A substantial body of research (e.g., Bandura et al., 1987; Dolce et al., 1986; Litt, 1988; Stevens et al., 2000; Williams & Kinney, 1991) indicates that people with low self-efficacy do not tolerate pain well, report greater pain intensity, and experience more interference because of pain. Perceptions of diminished physical capacities and reduced efficacy for coping with pain may correspond to feelings of helplessness, reduced tolerance for pain, and a perpetuation of suffering (e.g., Lackner, Carosella, & Feuerstein, 1996), as well as very high levels of health care utilization that can fuel the lamentable tendency of some health professionals to take patient concerns about pain less seriously (e.g., Unruh, 1996).

Fortunately, self-efficacy can be enhanced through experiences of successful coping and formal treatment programs. For example, training in various strategies to cope with pain is associated with increases in self-efficacy and tolerance for pain (e.g., Holroyd et al., 1984; Williams & Kinney, 1991). Therefore, individuals with relatively low levels of physical self-efficacy and efficacy for coping with pain may benefit from interventions that enhance self-efficacy, especially in the face of ongoing, benign pain.

With reference to coping, men in the sample were likely to divert attention away from CPT (e.g., by thinking about neutral or pleasant events), whereas women more often reinterpreted painful sensations (e.g., by redefining feelings of pain as numbness).

These findings are somewhat consistent with conclusions of recent literature reviews (e.g., Rollman et al., 2000; Unruh, 1996), which suggest that women more typically use emotion-focused or interpersonal—communal coping strategies (e.g., venting emotions, redefinition, catastrophizing, seeking spiritual comfort, and seeking emotional support), whereas men prefer strategies such as problem-focused coping, talking problems down, denial, and looking on the bright side. Given that diverting attention away from pain was associated with increased pain tolerance, the differential use of distraction might also have contributed to gender differences in pain perception.

It should be noted, however, that by its very nature, experimental pain research may be biased against the use of communal and interpersonal coping strategies such as expressing emotion and seeking affiliation and support (e.g., Lyons & Sullivan, 1998; Sullivan et al., 2000; Taylor, 2002) often favored by women. For example, use of standardized instructions in this study (e.g., asking only for an SUDS rating and minimizing any other verbal or nonverbal communication during CPT) would presumably inhibit interpersonal coping.

Consequently, experimental designs themselves cannot be dismissed as an influence on gender differences in response to experimental pain. Incorporation and assessment of communal–interpersonal approaches to coping in experimental research may elucidate whether different strategies are more preferred by and beneficial for women and men. Assessment of interpersonal–communal coping may also have utility for understanding adjustment among patients with clinical pain conditions.

Despite its possible implications, the main limitations of this research must be acknowledged. First, although there are relatively consistent gender differences in pain perception, further investigation with other age and cultural groups, heterogeneous community samples, and clinical samples as well as with different types of experimental and day-to-day pain is needed to determine the generalizability and robustness of current findings beyond the sample population assessed in this research. Second, coping was assessed in a very general way with a single question and the classification of responses on the basis of their consistency with specific empirically derived pain-coping strategies. Although use of a standardized open-ended question may have reduced the tendency to endorse strategies read on a self-report scale but not actually used, future investigations that incorporate more sensitive, continuous measures of coping may identify more subtle gender differences in ways of coping with pain. Third, just prior to each CPT, ice water was circulated manually by the experimenters; however, circulation did not continue during the task. Given that water circulation was not continuous, we cannot completely rule out differential warming of water due to gender differences in arm mass.

Finally, although self-efficacy is a potential cognitive mediator of associations between gender and pain responses, from a biopsychosocial perspective (e.g., Melzack & Wall, 1965), a comprehensive understanding of pain and its mechanisms requires an appreciation for and integration of biological, psychological, and sociocultural processes. To avoid overly simplistic, reductionistic explanations of relations between gender and pain perception, future research should incorporate other potential mediators to account more fully for this association. However, to avoid spuriously high associations and misleading conclusions that can accompany evaluating the impact of a large number of variables, the selection of biological, affective, cognitive, motivational, and sociocultural factors that may contribute to this association is best guided by carefully developed and refined theory-guided approaches.

REFERENCES

Baker, S., & Kirsh, I. (1991). Cognitive mediators of pain perception and tolerance. *Journal of Personality and Social Psychology, 61,* 504–511.

Bandura, A. (1997). *Self-efficacy: The exercise of control.* New York: Freeman.

Bandura, A., O'Leary, A., Taylor, C., Gauthier, J., & Gossard, D. (1987). Perceived self-efficacy and pain control: Opiold and nonopiold mechanisms. *Journal of Personality and Social Psychology, 53,* 563–571.

Bendelow, G. (1993). Pain perceptions, emotions, and gender. *Sociology of Health and illness, 15,* 273–293.

Bussey, K., & Bandura, A. (1999). Social cognitive theory of gender development and differentiation. *Psychological Review, 106,* 676–713.

Darlington, R. B. (1990). *Regression and linear models.* New York: McGraw-Hill.

Dolce, J. J., Doleys, D., Raczynski, J., & Lassie, J. (1986). The role of self-efficacy expectancies in the prediction of pain tolerance. *Pain, 27,* 261–272.

Faull, C., & Nichol, A. R. (1986). Temperament and behaviour in six-year-olds with recurrent abdominal pain: A follow up. *Journal of Child Psychiatry and Allied Disciplines, 27,* 539–544.

Fillingim, R. B. (2000). *Sex, gender, and pain: Progress in pain research and management.* Seattle: International Association for the Study of Pain.

Gijsbers, K., & Niven, C. A. (1995). Women and the experience of pain. In C. A. Niven & D. Carroll (Eds.), *The health psychology of women* (pp. 43–57). Philadelphia: Harwood.

Godin, G., & Shephard, R. J. (1985). Gender differences in perceived physical self-efficacy among older individuals. *Perceptual and Motor Skills, 60,* 599–602.

Holroyd, K., Penzien, D., Hursey, K., Tobin, D., Rogers, L., et al. (1984). Change mechanisms in EMG biofeedback training: Cognitive changes underlying improvements in tension headache. *Journal of Consulting and Clinical Psychology, 52,* 1039–1053.

Jackson, T., Pope, L., Nagasaka, T., Fritch, A., Iezzi, T., & Lim, B. (2002). *The impact of threat appraisal on pain tolerance and coping.* Manuscript submitted for publication.

Keefe, F. J., Lefebyre, J. C., Egert, J. F., Affleck, G., Sullivan, M. J., & Caldwell, D. S. (2000). The relationship of gender to pain, pain behavior, and disability in osteoarthritis patients: The role of catastrophizing. *Pain, 87,* 325–334.

Lackner, J. M., Carosella, A., & Feuerstein, M. (1996). Pain expectancies, pain, and functional self-efficacy as determinants of disability in patients with chronic low back disorders. *Journal of Consulting and Clinical Psychology, 64,* 212–220.

Lautenbacher, S., Moeltner, A., & Strian, F. (1991). Psychophysical features of the transition from pure heat perception to heat pain perception. *Perception and Psychophysics, 52,* 685–690.

Lazarus, R. S. (1999). *Stress and emotion: A new synthesis.* New York: Springer.

Lester, N., Lefebre, J. C., & Keefe, F. J. (1994). Pain in young adults: I. Relationship to gender and family pain history. *Clinical Journal of Pain, 10,* 282–289.

Levine, F, & de Simone, L. (1991). The effects of experimenter gender on pain report in male and female subjects. *Pain, 44,* 69–72.

Litt, M. D. (1988). Self-efficacy and perceived control: Cognitive mediators of pain tolerance. *Journal of Personality and Social Psychology, 54,* 149–160.

Lyons, R., & Sullivan, M. (1998). Curbing loss in illness and disability: A relationship perspective. In J. H. Harvey (Ed.), *Perspectives on personal and interpersonal loss* (pp. 137–152). New York: Taylor and Francis.

Melzack, R., & Wall, P. (1965). Pain mechanisms—A new theory. *Science,* 150, 971–979.

Riley, J. L., Robinson, M. F, Wise, E. A., Myers, C. D., & Fillingim, R. B. (1998). Sex differences in the perception of noxious experimental stimuli: A meta-analysis. *Pain, 74,* 181–187.

Robinson, M. E., Riley, J. F, & Myers, C. D. (2000). Psychosocial contributions to sex-related differences in pain responses. In R. B. Fillingim (Ed.), *Sex, gender, and pain: Progress in pain research and management* (pp. 41–68). Seattle: International Association for the Study of Pain.

Rollman, G. B., Lautenbacher, S., & Jones, K. S. (2000). Sex and gender differences in responses to experimentally induced pain. In R. B. Fillingim (Ed.), *Sex, gender, and pain. Progress in pain research and management* (pp. 165–190). Seattle: International Association for the Study of Pain.

Rosenstiel, A., & Keefe, F. J. (1983). The use of coping strategies in chronic low back pain patients. Relationships to patient characteristics and current adjustment. *Pain, 17,* 33–44.

Ryckman, R. M., Robbins, M. A., Thornton, B., & Cantrell, P. (1982). Development and validation of a Physical Self-Efficacy Scale. *Journal of Personality and Social Psychology, 42,* 891–900.

Stevens, M. J., Ohlwein, A. L., & Catanzaro, S. J. (2000). Further evidence that self-efficacy predicts acute pain. *Imagination, Cognition, and Personality, 19,* 185–194.

Sullivan, M., Bishop, S., & Pivik, J. (1995). The Pain Catastrophizing Scale: Development and validation. *Psychological Assessment, 7,* 524–532.

Sullivan, M., Rouse, D., Bishop, S., & Johnston, S. (1997). Thought suppression, catastrophizing, and pain. *Cognitive Therapy and Research, 21,* 555–568.

Sullivan, M. J., Tripp, D. A., & Santor, D. (2000). *Gender differences in pain and pain behavior: The role of catastrophizing. Cognitive Therapy and Research, 24,* 121–134.

Taylor, S. E. (2002). *The tending instinct.* New York: Times Books.

Unruh, A. M. (1996). Gender variations in clinical pain experience. Pain, *65,* 123–167.

Weisenberg, M., Tepper, I., & Schwarzwald, J. (1995). Humor as a cognitive technique for increasing pain tolerance. *Pain, 63,* 207–212.

Williams, S. L., & Kinney, P. (1991). Performance and nonperformance strategies for coping with acute pain: The role of perceived self-efficacy, expected outcomes, and attention. *Cognitive Therapy and Research, 15,* 1–19.

Wittig, A. F., Duncan, S. L., & Schurr, K. T. (1987). The relationship of gender, gender-role endorsement, and perceived physical self-efficacy to sport competition anxiety. *Journal of Sport Behavior, 10,* 192–199.

DISCUSSION QUESTIONS

1. What was the hypothesis in this study?
2. How did they measure pain tolerance?
3. What did the researchers find?
4. Why do the authors believe that they found this pattern of results?
5. What are the implications of these findings for the experience of pain amongst men and women?

7

Acupuncture in Patients with Osteoarthritis of the Knee: A Randomised Trial

C. Becker-Witt, B. Brinkhaus, S. Jena, K. Linde, A. Streng, S. Wagenpfeil, J. Hummelsberger, H.U. Walther, D. Melchart, and S.N. Willich

ABSTRACT

Background: *Acupuncture is widely used by patients with chronic pain although there is little evidence of its effectiveness. We investigated the efficacy of acupuncture compared with minimal acupuncture and with no acupuncture in patients with osteoarthritis of the knee.*

Methods: *Patients with chronic osteoarthritis of the knee (Kellgren grade ≤ 2) were randomly assigned to acupuncture (n = 150), minimal acupuncture (superficial needling at non-acupuncture points; n = 76), or a waiting list control (n = 74). Specialised physicians, in 28 outpatient centres, administered acupuncture and minimal acupuncture in 12 sessions over 8 weeks. Patients completed standard questionnaires at baseline and after 8 weeks, 26 weeks, and 52 weeks. The primary outcome was the Western Ontario and McMaster Universities Osteoarthritis (WOMAC) index at the end of week 8 (adjusted for baseline score). All main analyses were by intention to treat.*

The Lancet, July 9, 2005 v366 i9480 p136(8)

"Acupuncture in Patients With Osteoarthritis of the Knee: A Randomised Trial" by C. Becker-Witt, B. Brinkhaus, S. Jena, K. Linde, A. Streng, S. Wagenpfeil, J. Hummelsberger, H.U. Walther, D. Melchart, and S.N. Willich. © 2005 The Lancet Publishing Group, a division of Elsevier Science Ltd.

Results: *294 patients were enrolled from March 6, 2002, to January 17, 2003; eight patients were lost to follow-up after randomisation, but were included in the final analysis. The mean baseline-adjusted WOMAC index at week 8 was 26.9 (SE 1.4) in the acupuncture group, 35.8 (1-9) in the minimal acupuncture group, and 49.6 (2.0) in the waiting list group (treatment difference acupuncture vs minimal acupuncture −8.8, [95% CI -13-5 to −4.2], p = 0.0002; acupuncture vs waiting list −22.7 [−27.5 to −17.9], p < 0.0001). After 52 weeks the difference between the acupuncture and minimal acupuncture groups was no longer significant (p = 0.08).*
Interpretation: *After 8 weeks of treatment, pain and joint function are improved more with acupuncture than with minimal acupuncture or no acupuncture in patients with osteoarthritis of the knee. However, this benefit decreases over time.*

INTRODUCTION

Osteoarthritis most frequently affects the knee joint. (1) Anti-inflammatory drugs used to treat the symptoms of this disorder are associated with various side-effects. (2) Furthermore, for patients for whom these drugs do not lead to an adequate response, replacement surgery is often recommended. (3) Patients with chronic pain are increasingly using acupuncture for pain relief. (4) There is some evidence that acupuncture can be effective in treating pain and dysfunction in patients with osteoarthritis of the knee. In a systematic review including seven randomised controlled trials with a total of 393 patients, acupuncture was more effective than sham acupuncture in reducing pain, whereas for joint function the results were inconclusive. (5) These previous studies, however, were based on small sample sizes and the follow-up period was never longer than 3 months.

We aimed to investigate the efficacy of acupuncture compared with minimal acupuncture and with no acupuncture in patients with pain and dysfunction due to osteoarthritis of the knee.

METHODS

Patients

Patients were included in our study if they were aged 50–75 years, had been diagnosed with osteoarthritis according to the American College of Rheumatology criteria, had documented radiological alterations in the knee joint of grade 2 or more according to Kellgren-Lawrence criteria, (6,7) had an average pain intensity of 40 or more on a 100 mm visual analogue scale in the 7 days before baseline assessment, and if they gave written informed consent. The exclusion criteria were one or more of the following: pain in the knee caused by inflammatory, malignant, or autoimmune disease; or other reasons for pain in the knee, such as serious valgus-defective or varus-defective position.

Patients were also excluded if they had had knee surgery, arthroscopy of the affected knee in the past year, chondroprotective or intra-articular injection in the past 4 months, systemic corticoid treatment or beginning of a new treatment for osteoarthritis in the past 4 weeks, local antiphlogistic treatment, acupuncture treatment during the past 12 months, or physiotherapy or other treatments for osteoarthritis knee pain (with the exception of nonsteroidal anti-inflammatory drugs) during the previous 4 weeks. Additional exclusion criteria were application for pension or disability benefits, serious acute or chronic organic disease or mental disorder, pregnancy or breastfeeding, and blood coagulation disorders or coagulation-inhibiting medication other than aspirin. Most participants were recruited through reports in local newspapers; a few patients spontaneously contacted trial centres. All study participants provided written informed consent and were insured according to the German law for medical products.

Procedures

Patients were randomly assigned to a treatment group stratified by centre in a 2 : 1 : 1 ratio (acupuncture: minimal acupuncture: waiting list) with a centralised telephone randomisation procedure (random list generated with Samp Size 2.0). The 2 : 1 : 1 ratio was used to help with recruitment and increase the compliance of trial physicians. Minimal acupuncture served as a sham intervention; the additional no acupuncture waiting list control was included since minimal acupuncture might not be a physiologically inert placebo. Patients in the acupuncture and minimal acupuncture groups were unaware of their treatment allocation. The total follow-up study period per patient was 52 weeks. The study was undertaken according to common guidelines for clinical trials (Declaration of Hetsinki, ICH-GCP including certification by an external audit). The study protocol was approved by the appropriate ethics review boards and has been described in detail elsewhere. (8)

Study interventions were developed in a consensus process with acupuncture experts and societies, and provided by physicians who were trained (at least 140 h) and experienced in acupuncture. Both the acupuncture and minimal acupuncture treatments consisted of 12 sessions of 30 min duration, administered over 8 weeks (usually two sessions per week for the first 4 weeks, followed by one session per week in the remaining 4 weeks). For patients with bilateral osteoarthritis in the acupuncture and the minimal acupuncture groups, both knees were needled with at least eight out often proposed points (at least 16 needles altogether), whereas for patients with unilateral osteoarthritis, the physician was able to choose unilateral or bilateral acupuncture. For unilateral acupuncture, the treatment had to be done with at least eight needles. Patients in the waiting list group did not receive acupuncture treatment for a period of 8 weeks, after which time they then also received acupuncture.

Acupuncture treatment was semi-standardised: all patients were treated with a selection of local and distant points chosen by the acupuncturists according to the principles of traditional Chinese medicine. Additional points included body acupuncture points, ear acupuncture points, and trigger points. Patients were treated by use of at least six local acupuncture points from the following selection: (9) stomach 34, 35, 36; spleen 9, 10; bladder 40; kidney 10; gall bladder 33, 34; liver 8; extraordinary points Heding, Xiyan. Additionally, physicians selected and needled at least two distant points from the following selection: spleen 4, 5, 6; stomach 6; bladder 20, 57, 58, 60, 62; kidney 3. Sterile disposable one-time needles had to be used, but physicians were able to choose the needle length and diameter. Physicians were instructed to achieve de qi (an irradiating feeling deemed to indicate effective needling) if possible, and needles were stimulated manually at least once during each session.

Minimal acupuncture treatment entailed superficial insertion of fine needles (20–40 mm in length) at predefined, distant non-acupuncture points. (8) These non-acupuncture points were not in the area of the knee, and the selection of at least eight out of ten points was left to the physician's discretion. Physicians were instructed to avoid manual stimulation of the needles and provocation of de qi in the minimal acupuncture treatment. In investigator meetings, all acupuncturists received training in the application of minimal acupuncture, which included a videotape and a brochure showing detailed information about the procedure.

Patients in the waiting list group did not receive acupuncture treatment for 8 weeks after randomisation; from week 9 they received 12 sessions of the acupuncture treatment described above. In all treatment groups, patients were allowed to treat osteoarthritis knee pain with oral non-steroidal anti-inflammatory drugs if necessary. The use of other pain treatments, such as drugs acting through the central nervous system, or corticosteroids, was not allowed.

Patients were informed about acupuncture and minimal acupuncture in the study as follows: "In this study, different types of acupuncture will be compared. One type is similar to the acupuncture treatment used in China. The other type does not follow these principles, but has also been associated with positive outcomes in clinical studies."

All patients completed standard questionnaires at baseline, and after 8 weeks, 26 weeks, and 52 weeks. The first questionnaire was distributed to the patients by the study physician and completed before the start of treatment (baseline). Patients sent their completed questionnaires to the study office in sealed envelopes. Follow-up questionnaires were sent to all patients by the study office. The primary outcome measure was the Western Ontario and McMasters Universities Osteoarthritis Index. (10,11) In cases of bilateral osteoarthritis, the knee defined at baseline as most painful was the one assessed throughout the entire study. Furthermore, the patient questionnaire included a modified version of the German Society for the Study of Pain survey,(12) which uses the German version of the pain disability index; (13) a scale for assessing emotional aspects of pain (Schmerzempfindungs-Skala [SES]); (14) the depression scale (Allgemeine Depressionsskala [ADS]); (15) and the German version of the SF-36 (16) (MOS36-item short form quality-of-life questionnaire) to assess health-related quality of life. Additionally, several questions on sociodemographic characteristics, numerical rating scales for pain intensity, questions about workdays lost, and global assessments were asked. The number of days with pain and medication were documented in a diary by the patients.

Blinding to treatment and the credibility of the treatment method were assessed by the patients with a credibility questionnaire (17) after the third acupuncture session. At the end of the study, patients were asked whether they thought they had received acupuncture following the principles of Chinese medicine or the other type of acupuncture. Physicians documented medical history, acupuncture treatment, serious adverse events, and side-effects for each session. Patients also reported side-effects at the end of week 8.

Statistical Analysis

Confirmatory tests of the primary outcome measure (WOMAC index at the end of week 8) and all main analyses (with SPSS 11.5) were based on the intention-to-treat population and used all available data. Sensitivity analyses were done for the primary outcome measure by replacing missing data with multiple imputations and last value carried forward by use of SOLAS 3.0 (Statistical Solutions, Cork, Ireland). For multiple imputation, the propensity score method was used with the main outcome as variable to impute. Five imputed datasets were generated in addition to the last value carried forward. An analysis of covariance, (18) with the main outcome WOMAC score at the end of week 8 as the dependent variable and baseline WOMAC score and treatment group as independent variables, was undertaken as primary analysis to account for potential baseline differences. Resulting baseline-adjusted treatment effects are given together with 95% CI and corresponding p values as well as means and standard errors (SE) of the primary outcome for each treatment group. The same analysis was done for all secondary parameters at the end of week 8.

The study was powered to detect a change of eight score points on the WOMAC Index (19) between the acupuncture and minimal acupuncture groups with 80% power on the basis of a SD of 17 score points and a two-sided significance level of 5%. Exploratory analyses (two-sided t tests and χ^2 tests for pairwise comparisons of groups without adjustment for multiple testing) were done for follow-up measurements. Because the waiting list group could not be compared directly with the two other groups after 26 weeks and 52 weeks, all subsequent data from this group were only analysed descriptively. Additionally, a per protocol analysis was done including only patients with no major protocol violations by the end of week 8.

Role of the Funding Source

The trial was initiated after a request from German health authorities (Federal Committee of Physicians and Social Health Insurance Companies, German

Federal Social Insurance Authority) and sponsored by German Social Health Insurance Companies. The health authorities had requested a randomised trial that included a sham control and a follow-up period of at least 6 months. All other decisions on study design, data collection, data analysis, data interpretation, and writing of the report were the complete responsibility of the researchers. The corresponding author had full access to all the data in the study and had final responsibility for the decision to submit for publication.

RESULTS

Between March 6, 2002, and January 17, 2003, about 1100 patients with osteoarthritis of the knee applied to participate in the study. Of 300 patients randomised six were excluded from the intention-to-treat population because no baseline data were available, and they did not receive the study intervention. All the remaining 294 patients treated in a total of 28 outpatient centres were included in the intention-to-treat population. Three patients in the acupuncture group (one planned operation, one car accident, one reason unclear) and three in the minimal acupuncture group (one moved to another town, two reason unclear) stopped the acupuncture treatment prematurely. After 8 weeks, data for the main efficacy analysis were available for 285 (97%) patients. The per-protocol analysis included 224 patients.

All patients had previously been treated with analgesics. 95 (32%) had received acupuncture in the past (8% for osteoarthritis) and 261 (88%) patients expected a substantial improvement from acupuncture treatment. Table 1 shows the baseline characteristics of patients in the three study groups.

Patients in the acupuncture group were treated with a mean of 17 (SD 8) needles and patients in the minimal acupuncture group with a mean of 12 (3) needles. The average duration of sessions was about 30 min in both groups. All patients in the acupuncture group were treated at local and distant points; additional points were used in 609 (35%) treatment sessions and trigger points in 246 (14%) treatment sessions. After three treatment sessions, patients rated the credibility of acupuncture and minimal acupuncture much the same and as very high, and at the end of the study most patients believed that they had received acupuncture following the principles of Chinese medicine (table 2).

Figure 3 [figure deleted] shows the development of the mean WOMAC index score. The mean baseline-adjusted WOMAC index at the end of week 8 was 26.9 (SE 1.4) in the acupuncture group compared with 35.8 (1·9) in the minimal acupuncture group and 49.6 (2.0) in the waiting list group (treatment difference: acupuncture us minimal acupuncture -8.8 [95% CI -13.5 to -4.2], p = 0. 0002; acupuncture vs waiting list -22-7 [-27.5 to -17.9], p < 0. 0001). Figure 4 [figure deleted] shows the treatment effect for individual patients categorised with respect to treatment group. The results were very similar if missing values were replaced and if baseline values were entered in the

TABLE 1   Baseline Characteristics of Intention-to-Treat Population

	Total (n = 294)	Acupuncture (n = 149)
Women	195 (66%)	105 (70%)
Men	99 (34%)	44 (30%)
Age (years)	64.0 (6.5)	64.5 (6.4)
Body–mass index	29.0 (5.0)	29.5 (4.8)
>10 years of school	43 (16%)	16 (11%)
Kellgren criteria		
Kellgren 0	1 (0.3%)	0
Kellgren 1	15 (5%)	6 (4%)
Kellgren 2	121 (41%)	52 (35%)
Kellgren 3	120 (41%)	66 (44%)
Kellgren 4	37 (13%)	25 (17%)
Duration of disease (years)	9.2 (7.9)	9.1 (8.5)
Days per month with pain	26.2 (6.5)	26.2 (6.5)
Osteoarthritis bilateral	224 (76%)	110 (74%)
Previous treatment		
Pharmaceutical intervention (past 6 months)	97 (33%)	43 (29%)
Physiotherapy (past 6 months)	45 (15%)	22 (15%)
Previous acupuncture treatment	23 (8%)	14 (9%)
Average pain (VAS)	65.3 (14.5)	64.9 (14.2)
WOMAC Index	51.4 (18.7)	50.8 (18.8)
Disability (PDI)	28.0 (13.2)	27.9 (14.2)
Physical health (SF–36) ★	29.7 (7.7)	30.0 (7.4)
Mental health (SF–36) ★	51.3 (12.0)	51.8 (12.1)
Pain affective (SES, t standard scores)	48.9 (9.1)	48.8 (9.3)
Pain sensoric (SES, t standard scores)	52.7 (9.9)	52.4 (9.5)
Depression (ADS, t standard scores)	51.2 (9.4)	51.2 (10.0)
	Minimal Acupuncture (n = 75)	**Waiting List (n = 70)**
Women	49 (65%)	41 (59%)
Men	26 (35%)	29 (41%)
Age (years)	63.4 (6.6)	63.6 (6.7)
Body–mass index	28.8 (4.6)	28.3 (5.89)
>10 years of school	11 (17%)	16 (24%)
Kellgren criteria		
Kellgren 0	0	1 (1%)
Kellgren 1	5 (7%)	4 (6%)
Kellgren 2	29 (39%)	40 (57%)
Kellgren 3	32 (43%)	22 (31%)
Kellgren 4	9 (12%)	3 (4%)
Duration of disease (years)	9.9 (7.6)	8.8 (6.8)
Days per month with pain	26.6 (6.4)	25.7 (6.8)
Osteoarthritis bilateral	58 (77%)	56 (80%)

TABLE 1 *Continued*

	Minimal Acupuncture (n = 75)	Waiting List (n = 70)
Previous treatment		
Pharmaceutical intervention (past 6 months)	27 (36%)	27 (39%)
Physiotherapy (past 6 months)	7 (9%)	16 (23%)
Previous acupuncture treatment	5 (7%)	4 (6%)
Average pain (VAS)	68.5 (14.4)	62.8 (15.0)
WOMAC Index	52.5 (18.6)	51.6 (18.8)
Disability (PDI)	27.8 (13.2)	28.3 (11.3)
Physical health (SF-36) ★	29.2 (8.2)	29.8 (7.9)
Mental health (SF-36) ★	51.1 (11.6)	50.6 (12.1)
Pain affective (SES, t standard scores)	49.2 (8.7)	48.8 (9.3)
Pain sensoric (SES, t standard scores)	54.1 (10.8)	52.0 (10.0)
Depression (ADS, t standard scores)	51.3 (7.9)	51.2 (9.4)

Data are number (%) or mean (SD). WOMAC = questionnaire for assessing pain, function and stiffness due to osteoarthritis (Western Ontario and McMasters Universities Osteoarthritis Index); VAS = visual analogue scale; PDI = pain disability index; SF-36 = MOS 36-item short-form quality-of-life questionnaire; SES = questionnaire for assessing the emotional aspects of pain (Schmerzempfindungsskala); ADS = depression scale (Allgemeine Depressionsskala).

★ Higher values indicate better status.

TABLE 2 Treatment Credibility After the Third Treatment Session and Assessment of Blinding

	Acupuncture	Minimal Acupuncture	p
Credibility after third session	n = 148	n = 73	
Improvement expected	5.2 (1.1)	5.1 (0.9)	0.860
Recommendation to others	5.5 (1.0)	5.6 (0.7)	0.384
Treatment logical	5.0 (1.3)	4.8 (1.3)	0.327
Effective also for other diseases	5.6 (0.9)	5.7 (0.6)	0.601
Guess at end of week 52	n = 146	n = 71	0.332
"Chinese acupuncture"	96 (66%)	40 (56%)	
"The other type of acupuncture"	9 (6%)	4 (6%)	
"Don't know"	41 (28%)	27 (38%)	

Rating scale based on 0 = minimum and 6 = maximum agreement; data are number or mean (SD).

analysis of covariance as covariates. Additionally, the per-protocol analysis showed closely similar results.

Patients who received acupuncture had significantly better results for almost all secondary outcome measures than did those in the minimal acupuncture and waiting list groups. The proportion of responders (patients with a decrease of at least 50% in their WOMAC index score) was 52% in the acupuncture group compared with 28% in the minimal acupuncture group and 3% in the waiting list group (all patients with no data were counted as non-responders). On all WOMAC subscales (pain, stiffness, and physical function), the acupuncture group showed significant improvements compared with the minimal acupuncture and the waiting list groups (table 3). When weeks 1 and 8 were compared, the mean number of days per week with intake of analgesics decreased in the acupuncture group (from 1.4 [2.2] to 0.9 [2.0]) and in the minimal acupuncture group (from 1.5 [2.6] to 1.1 [2.3]), whereas in the waiting list control group this number remained closely similar (1.8 [2.3] vs 1.9 [2.6]). Additionally, the percentage of patients using analgesics in the acupuncture and minimal acupuncture groups decreased between weeks 1 and 8 (from 42% to 22% and from 38% to 23%, respectively), whereas in the waiting list group there was only a small change (from 52% to 45%). The improvements recorded after 8 weeks in the acupuncture and minimal acupuncture groups persisted during the follow-up period, although the differences between the groups were no longer significant after 26 or 52 weeks ($p = 0 - 063$ and 0.080 from exploratory analyses; table 4). The patients in the waiting list group who received acupuncture between weeks 9 and 16 showed improvements after treatment that were similar to those reported in the original acupuncture group (WOMAC index decreased from 51.6 [18.8] to 31.6 [20.6]).

During the 26 weeks after randomisation, a total of nine serious adverse events (three acupuncture, two minimal acupuncture, four waiting list) were documented. One patient from the minimal acupuncture group died from myocardial infarction. All cases were admitted to hospital and regarded as unrelated to the study condition or the intervention. 24 side-effects were reported by 20 (14%) patients in the acupuncture group (18 small haematoma or bleeding and six other side-effects, such as needling pain), and 16 side-effects by 13 (18%) patients ($p = 0.410$) in the minimal acupuncture group (nine small haematoma or bleeding, one case of local inflammation at the needling site, and six other side-effects).

DISCUSSION

In this study, patients with osteoarthritis of the knee who received acupuncture had significantly less pain and better function after 8 weeks than did patients who received minimal acupuncture or no acupuncture. After 26 and 52 weeks, exploratory analysis indicated that the differences between acupuncture and minimal acupuncture were no longer significant.

The present study is, to date, one of the largest and most rigorous trials of the efficacy of acupuncture available. Its strengths include a prepublished protocol, (8) interventions based on expert consensus by qualified and experienced medical acupuncturists, assessment of the credibility of interventions,

TABLE 3 Primary and Secondary Outcomes at the End of Week 8

Primary Outcome	Acupuncture Mean (SE)	Minimal Acupuncture Mean (SE)
Questionnaire		
WOMAC Index	26.9 (1.4)	35.8 (1.9)
WOMAC Pain	24.4 (1.4)	33.2 (2.0)
WOMAC Stiffness	32.7 (1.9)	42.3 (2.7)
WOMAC Physical function	27.0 (1.4)	35.8 (2.0)
Disability (PDI)	16.4 (0.9)	22.2 (1.2)
Physical health (SF-36) (†)	36.2 (0.6)	33.1 (0.8)
Mental health (SF-36) (†)	53.6 (0.7)	51.9 (1.0)
Pain affective (SES, t standard scores)	42.4 (0.7)	44.1 (0.9)
Pain sensoric (SES, t standard scores)	47.3 (0.7)	48.1 (1.0)
Depression		
(ADS, t standard scores)	47.9 (0.8)	48.3 (1.1)
Days with limited function	16.3 (1.5)	21.3 (2.1)
Diary		
Days with pain in week 8 (diary)	4.4 (0.2)	5.3 (0.3)
Days with medication in weeks 5-8 (diary)	4.5 (0.5)	4.6 (0.6)

	Waiting List Mean (SE)	Acupuncture vs Minimal Acupuncture* (95% CI)
Questionnaire		
WOMAC Index	49.6 (2.0)	−8.8 (−13.5 to −4.2)
WOMAC Pain	44.9 (2.1)	−8.8 (−13.7 to −3.9)
WOMAC Stiffness	55.0 (2.8)	−9.6 (−16.0 to −3.2)
WOMAC Physical function	50.4 (2.1)	−8.9 (−13.7 to −4.0)
Disability (PDI)	27.4 (1.3)	−5.8 (−8.8 to −2.8)
Physical health (SF-36) (†)	31.8 (0.9)	3.1 (1.1 to 5.1)
Mental health (SF-36) (†)	50.7 (1.0)	1.7 (−0.6 to 4.0)
Pain affective (SES, t standard scores)	5.9 (1.0)	−1.7 (−3.9 to 0.5)
Pain sensoric (SES, t standard scores)	49.8 (1.0)	−0.8 (−3.2 to 1.6)
Depression (ADS, t standard scores)	49.4 (1.1)	−0.5 (−3.1 to 2.1)
Days with limited function	27.4 (2.2)	−4.9 (−10.1 to 0.2)
Diary		
Days with pain in week 8 (diary)	6.4 (0.3)	−1.0 (−1.6 to −0.3)
Days with medication in weeks 5-8 (diary)	5.8 (0.7)	−0.1 (−1.6 to 1.5)

Continued

TABLE 3 *Continued*

Questionnaire	p	Acupuncture vs waiting list(95% CI)	p*
WOMAC Index	<0.001	−22.7 (−27.5 to −17.9)	<0.001
WOMAC Pain	<0.001	−20.5 (−25.5 to −15.5)	<0.001
WOMAC Stiffness	0.003	−22.3 (−28.9 to −15.7)	<0.001
WOMAC Physical function	<0.001	−11.0 (−28.4 to −18.4)	<0.001
Disability (PDI)	<0.001	−11.0 (−14.1 to −7.9)	<0.001
Physical health (SF-36) ([†])	0.003	4.4 (2.3 to 6.5)	<0.001
Mental health (SF-36) ([†])	0.137	2.9 (0.6 to 5.3)	0.016
Pain affective (SES, t standard scores)	0.134	−3.5 (−5.8 to −1.2)	0.003
Pain sensoric (SES, t standard scores)	0.494	−2.5 (−5.0 to −0.1)	0.044
Depression (ADS, t standard scores)	0.725	−1.5 (−4.1 to 1.1)	0.250
Days with limited function	0.059	−11.1 (−16.3 to −5.8)	<0.001
Diary			
Days with pain in week 8 (diary)	0.005	−2.1 (−2.8 to −1.4)	<0.001
Days with medication in weeks 5-8 (diary)	0.922	−1.3 (−3.0 to 0.3)	0.110

WOMAC=questionnaire for assessing pain, function, and stiffness due to osteoarthritis (Western Ontario and McMasters Universities Osteoarthritis Index); PDI=pain disability index; SF-36=MOS 36-item short-form quality-of-life questionnaire; SES=questionnaire for assessing the emotional aspects of pain (Schmerzempfindungsskala);ADS=depression scale (Allgemeine Depressionsskala).
* Mean baseline-adjusted treatment difference between groups.
([†]) Higher values indicate better status

outcome measurements as recommended in guidelines for trials on osteoarthritis, (20,21) and very high follow-up rates. One potential limitation of the study is that participants were recruited primarily through newspaper articles and might not be representative of all patients with osteoarthritis of the knee. Also, due to the nature of the intervention, it was not possible to blind acupuncturists to treatment. However, the primary outcome measure and all secondary outcome measures were assessed by the patients themselves. Acupuncture and minimal acupuncture are not strictly indistinguishable. One could, therefore, argue that our results might have been biased by a lack of sufficient blinding. Although this bias cannot be ruled out, a major bias seems unlikely to us for two reasons. First, patients were informed in a manner suggesting that two different types of acupuncture treatment were compared, not mentioning terms such as "placebo" or "sham." Similar strategies of informed consent have been used in most previous acupuncture trials. (22) Second, both acupuncture and minimal acupuncture were thought to be highly credible and most patients believed that they had received the Chinese acupuncture.

Compared with both waiting list control and minimal acupuncture, the effect of acupuncture on the WOMAC scale after 8 weeks is clinically

TABLE 4   Secondary Outcomes After 26 Weeks and 52 Weeks

At 26 weeks

	Acupuncture Mean (SD)	Minimal Acupuncture Mean (SD)
Questionnaire		
WOMAC Index	30.4 (21.3)	36.3 (22.3)
WOMAC Pain	28.9 (22.7)	33.8 (22.3)
WOMAC Stiffness	34.7 (25.3)	40.3 (26.1)
WOMAC Physical function	30.4 (21.4)	36.5 (23.2)
Disability (PDI)	18.6 (13.0)	22.8 (15.3)
Physical health (SF-36)[†]	35.1 (8.8)	33.0 (10.0)
Mental health (SF-36)[†]	52.6 (11.5)	51.7 (11.2)
Pain affective (SES, t standard scores)	41.3 (9.3)	43.4 (9.4)
Pain sensoric (SES, t standard scores)	46.0 (9.2)	48.0 (9.3)
Depression (ADS, t standard scores)	48.2 (9.9)	48.7 (9.3)
Days with limited function	41.8 (45.6)	61.1 (61.7)

At 26 weeks

	Acupuncture vs Minimal Acupuncture* (95%CI)	p
Questionnaire		
WOMAC Index	−5.8 (−12.0 to 0.3)	0.063
WOMAC Pain	−4.8 (−11.2 to 1.6)	0.137
WOMAC Stiffness	−5.6 (−12.8 to 1.7)	0.131
WOMAC Physical function	−6.2 (−12.4 to 0.1)	0.053
Disability (PDI)	−4.2 (−8.3 to −0.0)	0.048
Physical health (SF-36)[†]	2.1 (−0.5 to 4.8)	0.111
Mental health (SF-36)[†]	0.9 (−2.3 to 4.2)	0.580
Pain affective (SES, t standard scores)	−2.1 (−4.8 to 0.6)	0.120
Pain sensoric (SES, t standard scores)	−2.0 (−4.6 to 0.6)	0.138
Depression (ADS, t standard scores)	−0.5 (−3.6 to 2.5)	0.730
Days with limited function	−19.4 (−35.5 to −3.2)	0.019

At 52 weeks

	Acupuncture Mean (SD)	Minimal Acupuncture Mean (SD)
Questionnaire		
WOMAC Index	32.7 (22.4)	38.4 (22.6)
WOMAC Pain	30.0 (23.5)	33.5 (21.3)
WOMAC Stiffness	37.4 (25.2)	47.1 (28.0)
WOMAC Physical function	33.0 (23.0)	38.9 (23.8)
Disability (PDI)	20.0 (14.0)	23.6 (15.0)
Physical health (SF-36)[†]	5.0 (10.0)	32.8 (9.5)

Continued

TABLE 4 *Continued*

At 52 weeks

	Acupuncture Mean (SD)	Minimal Acupuncture Mean (SD)
Questionnaire		
Mental health (SF-36)[†]	52.9 (11.0)	51.1 (11.7)
Pain affective (SES, t standard scores)	42.5 (10.2)	44.1 (10.4)
Pain sensoric (SES, t standard scores)	47.7 (11.3)	48.4 (10.5)
Depression (ADS, t standard scores)	48.6 (10.2)	49.8 (10.1)
Days with limited function	41.1 (56.5)	67.8 (71.7)

At 52 weeks

	Acupuncture vs Minimal Acupuncture* (95% CI)	p
Questionnaire		
WOMAC Index	−5.7 (−12.1 to 0.7)	0.080
WOMAC Pain	−3.5 (−10.0 to 3.0)	0.285
WOMAC Stiffness	−9.7 (−17.1 to −2.2)	0.011
WOMAC Physical function	−5.9 (−12.5 to 0.7)	0.081
Disability (PDI)	−3.6 (−7.7 to 0.5)	0.089
Physical health (SF-36)[†]	2.2 (−0.6 to 5.1)	0.120
Mental health (SF-36)[†]	1.9 (−1.3 to 5.1)	0.254
Pain affective (SES, t standard scores)	−1.6 (−4.6 to 1.4)	0.291
Pain sensoric (SES, t standard scores)	−0.7 (−3.9 to 2.4)	0.643
Depression (ADS, t standard scores)	−1.2 (−4.3 to 1.8)	0.430
Days with limited function	−26.7 (−46.0 to −7.5)	0.007

WOMAC=Western Ontario and McMasters Universities Osteoarthritis Index; PDI = pain disability index; SF-36=MOS 36-item short-form quality-of-life questionnaire; SES=Schmerzempfindungsskala; ADS=Allgemeine Depressionsskala.

* Mean difference between groups; minor discrepancies between differences calculated from group means presented in the table are due to rounding.

[†] Higher values indicate better status.

important. (22) Significant differences were also evident for secondary outcomes. The differences between the acupuncture and the minimal acupuncture groups can probably not be explained by the intake of analgesics, which was much the same in both groups. Days with intake of analgesics did not differ between the acupuncture and minimal acupuncture groups, but differences cannot be ruled out completely because only days with intake of analgesics and not the exact number of pills or the dosage of analgesics was assessed. Exploratory analysis at 26 and 52 weeks' follow-up indicated that differences between acupuncture and minimal acupuncture were no longer significant.

Because the waiting list patients received acupuncture after 8 weeks, whether the benefit of acupuncture over no treatment is still clinically relevant in the long term is difficult to assess. In any case, our results suggest that a single course of acupuncture treatment has only limited long-term point-specific effects.

In this study, the side-effects of acupuncture were of only minor severity. Several large surveys have also provided evidence that acupuncture is a relatively safe treatment. (23–25) Non-steroidal anti-inflammatory drugs, which are the most common pharmaceutical treatment in patients with osteoarthritis, are well known for producing severe side-effects, such as gastrointestinal bleeding, causing many deaths. (2) A reduction in the use of non-steroidal anti-inflammatory drugs might be a potential secondary benefit of acupuncture treatment. Our results lend support to the findings of three previous smaller trials that compared acupuncture with a no-treatment control, two of which were randomised (26,27) and one was not. (28) Four published trials have compared acupuncture and sham acupuncture interventions. (29–32) In three of these trials, (30–32) pain improved significantly after treatment with acupuncture compared with sham acupuncture, whereas only one trial (32) reported a difference for function. In the trial that showed no difference between acupuncture and sham acupuncture, (29) acupuncture treatment was administered over a short period (three times a week for 3 weeks). One method of sham acupuncture is the minimum sham method (superficial needling at distant non-acupuncture points), which tries to keep to a minimum the nonspecific needling effects. (33) In our study, and in both trials with positive results, sham acupuncture was administered as minimum sham. In the third trial with neutral results, sham acupuncture was administered superficially, but near to the real acupuncture points. This procedure could have produced more analgesic effects than the method used in the other trials. The differences in findings with respect to function might be due to low statistical power in the early trials, use of different measurement instruments, or the possibility that our form of acupuncture treatment (using more local acupuncture points) was more effective in improving physical function in patients with osteoarthritis of the knee.

Most previous studies have included only a short-term follow-up. Only in the study by Molsberger and colleagues (30) was follow-up assessed at 3 months, yielding results that were similar to those immediately after treatment completion. However, in our study the outcome differences between acupuncture and minimal acupuncture treatment decreased during the 12-month follow-up period.

In conclusion, acupuncture treatment had significant and clinically relevant short-term effects when compared to minimal acupuncture or no acupuncture treatment in patients with osteoarthritis of the knee. We now need to assess the long-term effects of acupuncture, both in comparison to sham interventions and to standard treatment.

REFERENCES

1. Creamer P, Hochberg MC. Osteoarthritis. *Lancet* 1997; 350: 503–09.

2. Tramer MR, Moore RA, Reynolds DJ, McQuay HJ. Quantitative estimation of rare adverse events which follow a biological progression: a new model applied to chronic NSAID use. *Pain* 2000; 85: 169–82.

3. Anon. Recommendations for the medical management of osteoarthritis of the hip and knee: 2000 update. American College of Rheumatology Subcommittee on Osteoarthritis Guidelines. *Arthritis Rheum* 2000; 43: 1905–15.

4. Eisenberg DM, Davis RB, Ettner SL, et al. Trends in alternative medicine use in the United States, 1990-1997: results of a follow-up national survey. *JAMA* 1998; 280: 1569–75.

5. Ezzo J, Hadhazy V, Birch S, et al. Acupuncture for osteoarthritis of the knee: a systematic review. *Arthritis Rheum* 2001; 44: 819–25.

6. Kellgren JH. Radiolocical Assessment of Osteo-Arthrosis. *Ann Rheum Dis* 1957; 16: 494–502.

7. Kessler S, Guenther KP, Puhl W. Scoring prevalence and severity in gonarthritis: the suitability of the Kellgren & Lawrence scale. *Clin Rheumatol* 1998; 17: 205–09.

8. Brinkhaus B, Becker-Witt C, Jena S, et al. Acupuncture Randomized Trials (ART) in patients with chronic low back pain and osteoarthritis of the knee: design and protocols. *Forsch Komplementarmed Klass Naturheilkd* 2003; 10: 185–91.

9. Deadman P, Al-Khafaji M. *A manual of acupuncture.* Sussex, UK: Journal of Chinese Medicine Publications, 2001.

10. Bellamy N, Buchanan WW, Goldsmith CH, Campbell J, Stitt LW. Validation study of WOMAC: a health status instrument for measuring clinically important patient relevant outcomes to antirheumatic drug therapy in patients with osteoarthritis of the hip or knee. *J Rheumatol* 1988; 15: 1833–40.

11. Stucki G, Meier D, Stucki S, et al. Evaluation of a German version of WOMAC (Western Ontario and McMaster Universities) Arthrosis Index. *Z Rheumatol* 1996; 55: 40–49.

12. Nagel B, Gerbershagen HU, Lindena G, Pfingsten M. Entwicklung und empirische Uberprufung des Deutschen Schmerzfragebogens der DGSS. *Schmerz* 2002; 16: 263–70.

13. Dillmann U, Nilges P, Saile H, Gerbershagen HU. Behinderungseinschatzung bei chronischen Schmerzpatienten. *Schmerz* 1994; 100–10.

14. Geissner ESA. Die Schmerzempfindungsskala (SES). Gottingen: Hogrefe, 1996.

15. Hautzinger M, Bailer M. Allgemeine Depressionsskala (ADS). Die deutsche Version des CES-D. Weinheim: Beltz, 1993.

16. Bullinger M, Kirchberger I. SF-36 Fragebogen zum Gesundheitszustand. Gottingen: Hogrefe, 1998.

17. Vincent C. Credibility assessments in trials of acupuncture. *Complement Med Res* 1990; 4: 8–11.

18. Vickers AJ, Altman DG. Statistics notes: Analysing controlled trials with baseline and follow up measurements. *BMJ* 2001; 323: 1123–24.

19. Berman BM, Singh BB, Lao L, et al. A randomized trial of acupuncture as an adjunctive therapy in osteoarthritis of the knee. *Rheumatology* (Oxford) 1999; 38: 346–54.

20. Altman R, Brandt K, Hochberg M, et al. Design and conduct of clinical trials in patients with osteoarthritis: recommendations from a task force of the Osteoarthritis Research Society. Results from a workshop. *Osteoarthritis Cartilage* 1996; 4: 217–43.

21. Bellamy N, Kirwan J, Boers M, et al. Recommendations for a core set of outcome measures for future phase III clinical trials in knee, hip, and hand osteoarthritis. Consensus development at OMERACT III. *J Rheumatol* 1997; 24: 799–802.

22. Linde K, Dincer F. How informed is consent in sham-controlled trials of acupuncture? *J Altern Complement Med* 2004; 10: 379–85.

23. White AR, Hayhoe S, Hart A, Ernst E. Survey of Adverse events following Acupuncture (SAFA): a prospective study of 32 000 consultations. Department of Complementary Medicine, University of Exeter, Exeter, UK, 2001: 1–20.

24. Melchart D, Weidenhammer W, Streng A, et al. Prospective investigation of adverse effects of acupuncture in 97733 patients. *Arch Intern Med* 2004; 164: 104–05.

25. Yamashita H, Tsukayama H, Hori N, Kimura T, Tanno Y. Incidence of adverse reactions associated with acupuncture. *J Altern Complement Med* 2000; 6: 345–50.

26. Berman BM, Singh BB, Lao L, et al. A randomized trial of acupuncture as an adjunctive therapy in osteoarthritis of the knee. *Rheumatology* (Oxford) 1999; 38: 346–54.

27. Christensen BV, Luhl IU, Vilbek H, Bulow HH, Dreijer NC, Rasmussen HF. Acupuncture treatment of severe knee osteoarthrosis: a long-term study. *Acta Anaesthesiol Scand* 1992; 36: 519–25.

28. Tillu A, Tillu S, Vowler S. Effect of acupuncture on knee function in advanced osteoarthritis of the knee: a prospective, non-randomised controlled study. *Acupunct Med* 2002; 20: 19–21.

29. Takeda W, Wessel J. Acupuncture for the treatment of pain of osteoarthritic knees. *Arthritis Care Res* 1994; 7: 118–22.

30. Molsberger A, Bowing G, Jensen KU, Lorek M. Schmerztherapie mit Akupunktur bei Gonarthrose. *Der Schmerz* 1994; 8: 3742.

31. Petrou P, Winkler V, Genti G, Balint G. Double blind trial to evaluate the effect of acupuncture treatment on knee osteoarthritis. *Scand J Acupunct* 1988; 3: 112–15.

32. Sangdee C, Teekachunhatean S, Sananpanich K, et al. Electroacupuncture versus diclofenac in symptomatic treatment of osteoarthritis of the knee: a randomized controlled trial. *BMC Complement Altern Meal* 2002; 2: 3.

33. Vincent C, Lewith G. Placebo controls for acupuncture studies. *J R Soc Med* 1995; 88: 199–202.

DISCUSSION QUESTIONS

1. What was the purpose of this study?

2. What was the difference between acupuncture treatment and minimal acupuncture treatment in this study?

3. What did the researchers find? Did acupuncture reduce pain for patients with osteoarthritis of the knee?

4. What was one limitation of this study?

8

Results of a Heart Disease Risk-Factor Screening Among Traditional College Students

Leslie Spencer

ABSTRACT

The author collected data on serum cholesterol, blood pressure, and self-reported health behavior in 226 college students aged 18 to 26 years. Twenty-nine percent had undesirable total cholesterol levels, 10% had high cholesterol, 10% had high systolic blood pressure, and 11% had high diastolic blood pressure. Half or more of the participants consumed a diet high in saturated fats, engaged in binge drinking, had a parental risk for high cholesterol or blood pressure, or reported they experienced elevated stress levels. Men had higher risk-factor levels than women. Findings from a regression analysis revealed that smoking, binge drinking, lack of cardiovascular exercise, and eating a high saturated-fat diet were predictive of undesirable cholesterol levels. Study limitations included self-selection of participants and single measurements of blood pressure and cholesterol. Trained students served as screeners in the program for providing an effective, low-cost screening intervention.

Journal of American College Health, May 2002 v50 i6 p291(6)
"Results of a Heart Disease Risk-Factor Screening Among Traditional College Students"
by Leslie Spencer. © 2002 Heldref Publications

INTRODUCTION

Heart disease, the leading cause of death in the United States, accounted for 31.4% of all deaths in 1997. Although often considered a disease of middle age, heart disease is the third leading cause of death among adults aged 25 to 44 years and accounted for more than 16,000 deaths in this age group in 1997. (1) Because many risk factors for heart disease may begin in adolescence, national health organizations have targeted adolescents and young adults for prevention efforts. (1–3) Risk factors include tobacco use, hypertension, high blood cholesterol (with unfavorable low-density lipoprotein [LDL] and high-density lipoprotein [HDL] ratios), sedentary lifestyle, high-fat diets, excessive alcohol consumption, and high stress levels related to hypertension. (2–5)

Young adults who maintain low-risk lifestyles over time are significantly less likely to die prematurely from heart disease. (6–8) The Bogalusa Heart Study (9) reported that early-stage atherosclerosis in young people (ages 2–39 y) was directly related to the number of cardiovascular risk factors they possessed. The Pathobiological Determinants of Atherosclerosis in Youth (PDAY) Study (10) offered "compelling support" for beginning cardiovascular risk-factor prevention in childhood. The following are some of the heart disease risk-factor rates among young adults that were identified by the US Department of Health and Human Services in 1997 in Healthy People 2010:

- Tobacco use among adolescents increased during the 1990s and was highest among Whites, with 40% of all adolescents reporting that they currently smoked cigarettes.
- Binge drinking rates continued to climb, reaching an all-time high of 32% among individuals aged 18 to 25, who reported they consumed five or more drinks at one sitting.
- Overweight and obesity among adolescents and young adults also increased, with 11% of those under age 20 and 23% of those aged 20 or older considered to be overweight or obese.
- Only 15% of adults aged 18 and older exercised at recommended levels, and 40% were completely inactive. (1)

The National Cholesterol Education Program (NCEP) reported clear evidence that elevated blood cholesterol, a primary risk factor for atherosclerosis, begins in childhood. Children and adolescents with high blood cholesterol levels, the NCEP report continued, are more likely to develop heart disease as adults. (2) Recommended preventive practices include limiting saturated fats to no more than 10% of daily calories, total fat to no more than 30% of daily calories, and dietary cholesterol to no more than 300 mg per day. Total cholesterol of less than 200 mg/dL, LDL levels below 110 mg/dL, and HDL levels of 35 mg/dL or above are considered desirable. (11, 12) Revised guidelines, issued in May 2001, recommended LDL levels below 100 mg/dL and HDL levels above 40 mg/dL. (13)

The age at which serum cholesterol screening should begin is controversial. The NCEP recommends blood cholesterol screening every 5 years for all adults aged 20 years or older. (2) Stamler and colleagues (14) offer overwhelming support for this position, citing the results of three large prospective studies that indicate a strong, clear, and direct relationship between high serum cholesterol in young adulthood and premature death from coronary heart disease (CHD). Rifai and associates (15) support this view, expressing fear that selective screening among young adults is biased against minority groups and significantly reduces detection of high risks among African Americans. Reasons for delaying general population screening until age 25 or older include overemphasis on the importance of childhood cholesterol levels, (16) lack of evidence that treatment of elevated cholesterol levels in young adults leads to fewer CHD deaths, and the relatively low prevalence of high cholesterol in young adults. (17)

Overall rates of hypertension have leveled, and detection and treatment have increased over the past 2 decades for the 50 million Americans who had the disease in 1997, but 75% of those individuals did not receive adequate treatment. (3) Adults aged 18 and older should maintain a systolic blood pressure below 140 mm Hg and a diastolic blood pressure below 90 mm Hg. Systolic levels between 130 and 139 mm Hg are not diagnosed as high, yet a diastolic level between 85 and 90 is a concern because it may lead to hypertension and heart damage. (3, 18) Although detection and treatment of hypertension are important, primary prevention remains the ideal defense and should be initiated in young adulthood. (18) Preventive strategies include consuming a low-fat diet, maintaining a healthy weight, using no tobacco, restricting alcohol intake to two or fewer drinks per day, exercising regularly, and managing stress. (3, 19)

Colleges provide a unique opportunity to reach many young adults with CHD risk-reduction information. Various researchers have identified the poor health habits of college students, such as unhealthy diets, (20–26) lack of exercise, (21, 22, 24, 25) high stress, (21, 22–27) tobacco use, (25, 28–31) and excessive alcohol consumption. (32–36) Even when students indicate they know a lot about cardiovascular risks, their behaviors often do not reflect their knowledge. (25) Less is known about traditional-aged college students' cholesterol levels. (37) In one of the few studies to offer descriptive norms of college students, Sparling and associates (38) found that 11% of the students they surveyed had elevated serum cholesterol levels.

My primary purpose in conducting this study was to provide normative data on CHD risk factors, including blood cholesterol and blood pressure, in a sample of traditional-aged college students. Published data for this population are sparse, and I found no studies that measured the risk factors I included in my research or explored the relationships among them. My secondary purpose was to describe a cost-effective, student-led, campus-wide heart disease risk-factor screening and counseling program. Such a comprehensive CHD risk-screening and counseling program requires materials, equipment, and trained staff that are not readily available in many educational settings. The program I describe was effective in providing an accurate assessment to participants at minimal expense because it used trained student volunteers to coordinate and perform the screening.

METHOD

The Program

I designed the program to provide accurate CHD risk-screening information and individualized recommendations for reducing risks in a single 20-minute session. I obtained approval from the University Institutional Review Board (IRB) before conducting the screening.

The portable screening facility is available during the academic year in various campus settings, including the health fair, lobbies in classroom and student services buildings, residence halls, and fraternity/sorority houses. Students volunteer to participate, and appointments are not necessary. A trained screener greets student participants, explains the procedure, and asks them to complete a written consent form and a risk-assessment survey. The screener briefly reviews the survey and engages the participant in conversation about his or her risk factors, and then uses an aneroid sphygmomanometer and stethoscope and a portable cholesterol analyzer (39) to check blood pressure and cholesterol levels.

The screener also draws several drops of blood from the participant's finger and applies the sample to a test strip. The test provides total cholesterol (TC) and high-density lipoprotein (HDL) measurements and the TC:HDL ratio. I decided not to test for low-density lipoprotein (LDL) because walk-in participants would have to fast in advance. In addition, elevated HDL is a significant risk factor and reducing HDL levels reduces the risk of CHD. (40) The TC:HDL ratio is also a useful measurement for determining whether the HDL is acceptable, compared with the overall TC level. (41) In addition, testing for LDL would add significantly to the cost of the test strips and was not within my budget. Once the tests are complete (approximately 10 minutes), the screener writes the results on an educational hand-out and explains them to the participant, with individualized suggestions for reducing heart disease risk in terms of the participant's survey and test results.

Data Collection

The Healthy Heart Screening program includes a brief written survey of participants' gender, age, ethnicity, heredity, tobacco use, diet, exercise, perceived stress level, alcohol consumption, blood pressure, and blood cholesterol readings.

Screeners are all sophomore through senior students in the health-promotion and fitness-management (HPFM) academic programs. To become a certified screener, the student must be enrolled in the Foundations of HPFM course, participate in a 4-hour practical training program, pass written and practical exams, and complete one screening under the close supervision of a trainer. Trainers are certified and experienced seniors who conduct the 4-hour practical training program, schedule the screenings, and supervise all screening events as the major project in their HPFM practicum. Each semester, the HPFM faculty identifies and supervises two or three trainers. The screeners also receive course credit for certification and participation in the program. By building the heart disease risk-factor screening program directly into the curriculum, faculty members can monitor its quality and ensure active student participation as screeners and trainers.

Participants

Two hundred twenty-six students (ages 18–26 y, M = 21) volunteered to participate in the program at an institution in southern New Jersey with an enrollment of approximately 10,000 students. Fifty-seven percent of the participants were women, and 84% were White. I collected data between January 2000 and May 2001.

Data Analysis

I used the chi-square test to identify significant differences between at-risk and low-risk participants in terms of gender, smoking status, and parental history of heart disease; correlations to explore the relationships among non-dichotomous variables; and multiple regression to identify the predictive value of the lifestyle variables (diet, smoking, exercise, alcohol consumption, and stress) for serum cholesterol and blood pressure. In addition, I used t tests to explore the mean differences in cholesterol and blood pressure that were related to gender, smoking status, and parental history of heart disease. Finally, I used analysis of variance (ANOVA) to identify mean differences in cholesterol and blood pressure related to the remaining lifestyle variables (diet, exercise, alcohol consumption, and stress). For data analysis, the Statistical Package for the Social Sciences (SPSS) version 10.0 was used.

RESULTS

Blood Pressure and Cholesterol Screening

I measured TC in 207 participants and found a range from 100 to 404 mg/dL (M = 185 mg/dL; SD = 39.65). When I defined 200 mg/dL or above as undesirable and 240 mg/dL or above as at risk, (2, 13) I found that 29% (n = 60) of the participants had undesirable TC and 7.7% (n = 16) were at risk. In the

112 participants for whom I measured HDL, the range was from 15 to 97 mg/dL (M = 56 mg/dL; SD = 16.92). I judged HDL below 35 mg/dL as at risk (12) and found that 10.7% (n = 12) of the participants fell into the at-risk category. Under the newer at-risk standard of below 40 mg/dL, (13) the percentage of at-risk participants rose to 18.7% (n = 21).

I calculated the TC:HDL ratio for 101 participants (not included in the initial screening) and found a range from 1.8 to 11.3 (M = 3.7; SD = 1.6). With the criteria of 6:1 or lower as desirable, 7.9% (n = 8) of the participants showed undesirable ratios. With 5:1 or lower as desirable and HDL recommended minimums increased to <40 mg/dL, 15.8% of the participants (n = 16) had undesirable ratios. Even if TC was above the desired range, a favorable ratio could be obtained if HDL was high enough, indicating less risk than if TC was high and HDL was low. Although lowering the TC level would still be ideal, it is not as great a concern as a ratio that is also at an undesirable level.

The screeners measured blood pressure in 122 participants. I considered at-risk levels of 140 mm systolic or higher or 90 mm diastolic or higher. Systolic blood pressure levels ranged between 70 and 199 (M = 122; SD = 17.23). Diastolic levels ranged from 50 to 130 (M = 76; SD = 11.98). Just over 10.5% of the participants (n = 13) showed at-risk systolic blood pressure levels, and 11.5% (n = 14) were at risk because of their diastolic blood pressure levels. With the criteria for undesirable blood pressure levels increased to include borderline systolic measures above 130 mm and diastolic measures above 85 mm, (3) the percentage of at-risk participants for systolic blood pressure increased to 21.3% (n = 26) and for diastolic blood pressure increased to 15.6% (n = 19). Note that screeners took but one blood pressure reading for each participant following a finger-stick blood draw for cholesterol. Had a follow-up reading been taken at another time, some participants' blood pressure might have been lower.

Self-Reported Measures

Analysis of the self-reported measures (completed by 226 participants) showed that 50% (n = 113) had at least one parent with high cholesterol or blood pressure. In addition, 14% (n = 32) of those students responded yes when asked whether they smoked. Fifty-seven percent of those students reported they smoked more than 20 cigarettes in a week, and 8 respondents, including 1 woman, indicated having used other forms of tobacco (pipes, cigars, or chewing tobacco).

Fifty-two percent (n = 116) of the students reported that they consumed two or more servings per day of foods high in saturated fats; of those, 6.6% (n = 15) ate five or more servings per day. In estimating their fiber intake, 33% (n = 75) of the respondents reported having less than two servings per day and 17% (n = 39) reported they had less than one serving per day. Of the 220 who responded to the question, "How many times per week do you perform cardiovascular exercise?" 36% (n = 80) reported two or fewer times a week, and 11% (n = 24) of the respondents said they exercised less than once a week.

Of the 154 participants who rated their stress levels, 4% (n = 9) called themselves "extremely stressed," 18% (n = 41) reported being "very stressed," and 32% (n = 72) said they were "moderately stressed."

Consuming 5 or more alcoholic drinks in 1 sitting is defined as binge drinking. (4) Forty-six percent (n = 70) of the 153 respondents said they "rarely or never" drank at the binge level, 22% (n = 34) drank that much once a month, and 14% (n = 21) did so once a week, whereas 18% (n = 28) responded that they drank 5 or more alcoholic drinks in one setting more than once a week.

Statistical Findings

I performed a chi-square test to determine whether gender, smoking status, or parental risk was related to participants' risk factors. Women were significantly less likely than men to eat diets that are high in saturated fats (χ^2 = 25.01, df = 3, p = .00) or binge drink (χ^2 = 20.83, df = 5, p = .001). Smokers were more likely than nonsmokers to have an unfavorable TC:HDL ratio of 6:1 or higher (χ^2 = 59.78, df = 42, p = .037) or to binge drink (χ^2 = 14.59, df = 5, p = .012). Participants who reported having at least 1 parent with high blood pressure or cholesterol were more likely to have a TC measure of 200 mg/dL or higher than participants whose parents had neither of these risks (χ^2 = 238.16, df = 202, p = .041).

Correlational analyses revealed the following important relationships between variables: significant positive relationships were apparent between consumption of high saturated-fat foods and TC:HDL ratio (r = .337, n = 100, p = .001); cardiovascular exercise and consumption of high fiber foods (r = .180, n = 220, p = .008); age and systolic blood pressure (r = .225, n = 122, p = .013); total cholesterol and diastolic blood pressure (r = .203, n = 107, p = .036); frequency of binge drinking and the TC:HDL ratio (r = .222, n = 98, p = .028); and frequency of binge drinking and consumption of high saturated-fat foods (r = .161, n = 152, p = .048).

By contrast, I found significant negative relationships between frequency of binge drinking and HDL level (r = −.194, n = 109, p = .043) and frequency of binge drinking and stress level (r = −.166, n = 153, p = .04). When I used the Pearson correlation, the relationship between the number of cigarettes smoked and total cholesterol level appeared to be a slightly significant negative relationship (r = −.376, n = 29, p = .044). This relationship was not confirmed when I used two nonparametric correlational tests; therefore these findings must be interpreted cautiously, given the small sample of smokers in the analysis.

I used stepwise multiple regression with the lifestyle and parental-risk variables to determine how well TC, HDL, TC:HDL ratio, and systolic and diastolic blood pressure could be predicted. A backward elimination approach

TABLE 1 Multiple Regression to Predict High-Lipoprotein Variables Used in Screening Heart Disease Factors Among Traditional College Students

Variable	Parameter	t	p
Intercept	69.415	7.957	.000**
Dietary fat	−.199	−2.122	.036 *
Exercise	.107	1.137	.258
Binge drinking	−.157	−1.67	.098
Smoking	−.166	−1.747	.084

$R^2 = .107$; $F = 3.079$, $p = .019$; * $p < .05$; ** $p < .001$.

TABLE 2 Multiple Regression to Predict the Total Cholesterol: High-Density Lipoprotein Ratio in Screening Heart Disease Factors Among Traditional College Students

Variable	Parameter	t	p
Intercept	1.531	2.425	.017*
Dietary fat	.354	3.751	.000**
Binge drinking	.196	2.071	.041*
Smoking	.132	1.391	.168

$R^2 = .182$; $F = 6.904$, $p = .000$; * $p < .05$; ** $p < .001$.

involved including all predictor variables in the equation and eliminating them one by one until only the most predictive remained. I found statistically significant regression models for HDL and TC:HDL ratio (see Tables 1 and 2). HDL levels were best predicted by smoking, cardiovascular exercise, binge drinking, and daily servings of high saturated-fat food, $F(4, 103) = 3.09$, $p = .02$. TC:HDL ratio was best predicted by smoking, binge drinking, and daily servings of foods high in saturated fats, $F(3, 93) = 6.90$, $p = .00$.

Next, I conducted independent t tests comparing the group means of total cholesterol, HDL, TC:HDL ratio, and systolic and diastolic blood pressure with gender. The mean HDL level for women was significantly higher than that for men ($t = 3.94$, $df = 110$, $p = .00$). The mean TC:HDL ratio ($t = 3.17$, $df = 99$, $p = .002$) and systolic blood pressure ($t = −2.016$, $df = 120$, $p = .046$) were significantly lower for women than for men. An independent t test comparing the group means of smokers and nonsmokers on these same variables showed that nonsmokers had significantly lower mean HDL levels ($t = −2.17$, $df = 17.29$, $p = .045$) than smokers. Again, given the small number of smokers, these results should be interpreted cautiously.

I used the ordinal lifestyle variables (diet, exercise, alcohol consumption, and stress) to perform several one-way analyses of variance (ANOVA) to detect mean differences in TC, HDL, TC:HDL ratio, and systolic and diastolic blood pressure as independent variables. Only the mean difference in TC:HDL ratio was significant, $F(3, 96) = 5.93$, $p = .001$. A Tukey HSD post hoc test revealed a significant mean difference in TC:HDL ratios between participants who consumed fewer than one serving of foods with high saturated fats per day and those who consumed 2 to 4 servings of high saturated-fat foods per day.

COMMENT

The following are some of my conclusions from this study of traditional-aged college students.

First, college students are at risk for heart disease; 29% of the participants had undesirable TC levels and up to 18% were above recommended levels for TC, HDL, and TC:HDL. They also were at risk for high blood pressure because approximately 15% to 21% had borderline levels; 10% to 11% were at risk for high systolic or diastolic blood pressure; half or more of all participants had at least one parent diagnosed with high cholesterol or blood pressure; they were under moderate to severe stress (54%); they consumed a diet high in saturated fats (52%); and they engaged in binge drinking at least once a month (52%). More than 30% did not consume adequate amounts of fiber or get enough cardiovascular exercise, and 14% were regular smokers.

Second, the students' unhealthy lifestyles were predictive of unfavorable serum cholesterol readings. Smoking, binge drinking, consuming a diet high in saturated fats, and being sedentary were significantly predictive of TC and HDL levels. Differences in the mean TC:HDL ratio were influenced by the number of servings of foods high in saturated fats (2–4 vs 1 or fewer) consumed daily. HDL levels decreased for participants as binge drinking increased.

Third, men in this population were particularly at risk; they were more likely than women to binge drink, to eat a diet high in saturated fats, and to have unfavorable blood pressure and TC levels and TC:HDL ratios.

Limitations

This research, although it points to some important preliminary findings, has several limitations. Self-selection bias is a concern because participants volunteered to participate in the screening. Although the reported smoking rate was low (14%), an earlier investigation of this campus population showed the smoking rate at 27%, (42) which suggested that students who participated in the screening might have had healthier habits than those who did not.

The screeners took measures only once for each student because of limited time and resources. A follow-up measure to confirm blood pressure and cholesterol readings would have increased their accuracy. The questionnaire contained only one survey inquiry to screen hereditary factors for CHD, and this limited the conclusions that one can draw about heredity and present risk in this population.

Future studies should use random sampling to verify these findings. A large-scale screening of randomly selected participants more representative of the campus population would yield a more complete and accurate assessment of CHD risks among young college adults. Some participants may have found having blood drawn for cholesterol testing stressful, and their stress might have caused an increase in blood pressure. (The screeners measured cholesterol first because it took 10 minutes to obtain a result; time limitations dictated the order of the screening.) A study in which blood pressure and cholesterol are measured at different times would eliminate this confounding effect. Future evaluation studies should also investigate the effect of behavior change programs on blood pressure and cholesterol in this population.

Although CHD disease may not manifest itself for several decades, these young-adult college students showed evidence of several cardiac risk factors. Many of the risks can be partially or wholly modified through changes in lifestyle. I conclude that a brief unscheduled screening and counseling intervention led by trained students is an effective, low-cost means of providing college students with information and education about CHD risk factors. Incorporating the program into an undergraduate health-promotion curriculum also provides excellent professional training and experience for health-promotion majors.

CHD begins to develop in young adulthood; in this study, I found preliminary evidence that college students have behavioral and biochemical risk factors favoring CHD. College health educators with limited resources can develop effective screening programs that use trained peer screener-educators and can build the screenings into the curriculum. Screening in conjunction with new or existing programs for behavior change in the areas of tobacco, diet, alcohol, stress, and exercise are an opportunity to measure how these programs can reduce risk factors for future heart disease.

REFERENCES

1. Healthy People 2010. Conference edition, 2 vols. US Department of Health and Human Services. Washington, DC: January 2000.

2. National Cholesterol Education Program. Report of the expert panel on blood cholesterol levels in children and adolescents. *Pediatrics*. 1992;89(suppl):525–584.

3. The Sixth Report of the Joint National Committee on Prevention, Detection, Evaluation, and Treatment of High Blood Pressure. *Arch Intern Med*. 1997;157:2413–2458.

4. Healthy People 2000: *National Health Promotion and Disease Prevention Objectives*. US Dept of Health and Human Services. DHHS publication no. (PHS) 91–50213.

5. Multiple Risk Factor Intervention Trial Research Group. *JAMA*. 1982; 248:1465–1477.

6. Stamler J, Stamler R, Neaton JD, et al. Low risk-factor profile and long-term cardiovascular and noncardiovascular mortality and life expectancy: Findings for 5 large cohorts of young adult and middle-aged men and women. *JAMA*. 1999;282:2012–2018.

7. Klag MJ, Ford DE, Mead LA, et al. Serum cholesterol in young men and subsequent cardiovascular disease. *N Engl J Med.* 1993;328:313–318.

8. Anderson KM, Castelli WP, Levy D. Cholesterol and mortality: 30 years of follow-up from the Framingham study. *JAMA.* 1987;257:2176–2180.

9. Berenson GS, Srinivasan SR, Bao W, et al. Association between multiple cardiovascular risk factors and atherosclerosis in children and young adults. *N Engl J Med.* 1998;338:1650–1655.

10. Strong JP, Malcom GT, McHahan CA, et al. Prevalence and extent of atherosclerosis in adolescents and young adults. *JAMA.* 1999;281:727–734.

11. Report of the National Cholesterol Education Program expert panel on detection, evaluation, and treatment of high blood cholesterol in adults. *Arch Intern Med.* 1988;148:36–69.

12. Summary of the second report of the National Cholesterol Education Program expert panel on detection, evaluation, and treatment of high blood cholesterol in adults (Adult Treatment Panel II). *JAMA.* 1993;269:3015–3023.

13. *Summary of the third report of the National Cholesterol Education Program expert panel on detection, evaluation, and treatment of high blood cholesterol in adults (Adult Treatment Panel III).* May 2001. National Institutes of Health publication 01–3670.

14. Stamler J, Daviglus M, Garside DB, et al. Relationship of baseline serum cholesterol levels in 3 large cohorts of younger men to long-term coronary, cardiovascular, and all-cause mortality and to longevity. *JAMA.* 2000;284:311–318.

15. Rifai N, Neufeld E, Ahlstrom P, et al. Failure of current guidelines for cholesterol screening in urban African American adolescents. *Pediatrics.* 1996;98:383–388.

16. Newman TB, Garber AM. Cholesterol screening in children and adolescents. *Pediatrics.* 2000;105:637–638.

17. Grundy S. Early detection of high cholesterol levels in young adults. *JAMA.* 2000;284:365–367.

18. McCarron P, Smith GD, Ohasha M, et al. Blood pressure in young adulthood and mortality from cardiovascular disease. *Lancet.* 2000;355:1430–1431.

19. Frazier L. Factors influencing blood pressure: Development of a risk model. *J Cardiovasc Nurs.* 2000;15:62–79.

20. Brevard PB, Ricketts CD. Residence of college students affects dietary intake, physical activity, and serum lipid levels. *J Am Diet Assn.* 1996;96(1):35–41.

21. Oleckno WA, Blacconiere MJ. Wellness of college students and differences by gender, race and class standing. *College Student Journal.* 1990a;24:421–429.

22. Makrides L, Veinot P, Gallivan T, et al. A cardiovascular health needs assessment of university students living in residence. *Can J Public Health.* 1988;89(3):171–175.

23. Troyer D, Ullrich IH, Yeater RA, et al. Physical activity and condition, dietary habits and serum lipids in second-year medical students. *J Am Coll Nutr.* 1990;9:303–307.

24. Glore SR, Walker C, Chandler A. Dietary habits of first-year medical students as determined by computer software analysis of the ie-day food records. *J Am Coll Nutr.* 1993;12:517–520.

25. Frost R. Cardiovascular risk modification in the college student: Knowledge, attitudes and behaviors. *J Gen Intern Med.* 1992;7:317–320.

26. Larouche R. Determinants of college students' health-promoting lifestyles. *Clinical Excellence for Nurse Practitioners.* 1998;2(1):35–44.

27. Lesko WA, Summerfield L. Academic stress and health changes in female college students. *Health Education.* 1989;20:18–21.

28. Emmons KM, Wechsler H, Dowdall G, et al. Predictors of smoking among US college students. *Am J Public Health*. 1998;88(1):104–107.

29. Sax LJ. Health trends among college freshmen. J Am Coll Health. 1997;45(6): 252–262.

30. Schorling JB, Gutgesell M, Las P, et al. Tobacco, alcohol and other drug use among college students. *J Subst Abuse*. 1994; 6:105–115.

31. Fiore MC, Jorenby DE, Wetter DW, et al. Prevalence of dally and experimental smoking among University of Wisconsin-Madison undergraduates. *WMJ*. 1993;92(11):605–608.

32. Wechsler H, Kuo M. College students define binge drinking and estimate its prevalence: Results of a national survey. *J Am Coll Health*. 2000;49(2):57–64.

33. Justus AN, Finn PR, Steinmetz JE. The influence of traits of disinhibition on the association between alcohol use and risky sexual behavior. *Alcoholism*. 2000;24(7):1028–1035.

34. Joly BM, McDermott RJ, Westhoff WW. Transportation practices of college students: Effects of gender and residential status on risk of injury. *International Electronic Journal of Health Education*. 2000;3(2):117–125.

35. Barrios LC, Everett SA, Simon TR, et al. Suicide ideation among US college students: Associations with other injury risk behaviors. *J Am Coll Health*. 2000;48(5):229–233.

36. Babor TF, Aguirre-Molina M, Marlatt GA, et al. Managing alcohol problems and risky drinking. *American Journal of Health Promotion*. 1999;14(2):98–103.

37. Brotons C, Ribera A, Perich RM, et al. Worldwide distribution of blood lipids and lipoproteins in childhood and adolescence: A review study. *Atherosclerosis*. 1998; 139:1–9.

38. Sparling PB, Snow TK, Beavers BD. Serum cholesterol levels in college students: Opportunities for education and intervention. *J Am Coll Health*. 1999;48(3):123–130.

39. *LDX Procedure Manual*. Cholestech Corporation, 3347 Hayward Blvd. Hayward, CA 94545–3808. Cholestech. 1996.

40. Grundy SM, Goodman DS, Rifkind BM, et al. The place of HDL in cholesterol management: A perspective from the national cholesterol education program. *Arch Intern Med*. 1989;149: 505–510.

41. Castelli WP, Abbott RID, McNamara PM. Summary estimates of cholesterol used to predict coronary heart disease. *Circulation*. 1983;67:730–734.

42. Spencer LS. College freshman smokers vs non-smokers: Academic, social and emotional expectations and attitudes toward college. *Journal of Health Education*. 1999;30(5):273–281.

DISCUSSION QUESTIONS

1. What is the purpose of this study?

2. Why is this an important study to conduct?

3. What did the researchers find? Summarize the results.

4. What are the implications of these findings for the health behavior of college students?

9

A Closer Look at Social Support as a Moderator of Stress in Breast Cancer

Cleora S. Roberts, Charles E. Cox, Vicki J. Shannon, and Nancy L. Wells

ABSTRACT

This study explored the effects of perceived social support from friends, family, and spouses on the psychological adjustment of 135 newly diagnosed breast cancer patients. Initial data analyses revealed moderate correlations between greater psychological distress and lower levels of social support. However, when the personality variable of social desirability was controlled for, the relationships between social support and well-being were substantially weakened or eliminated. It is concluded that characteristics of the person, rather than of the situation, underlie the apparent relationship between social support and adjustment to illness. Social workers are advised to make in-depth assessments of ego strengths and past psychological functioning as better predictors of patient adaptation to disease.

Introduction

Assessment of the social support networks available to patients coping with illness is generally accepted as an integral function of health care social work.

Health and Social Work, August 1994 v19 n3 p157(8)
"A Closer Look at Social Support as a Moderator of Stress in Breast Cancer" by Cleora S. Roberts, Charles E. Cox, Vicki J. Shannon, and Nancy L. Wells. © 1994 National Association of Social Workers

Knowledge of the impact, limitations, and mechanisms of social support for various patient populations leads to more accurate psychosocial assessments and, ultimately, better treatment plans.

The research study described in this article examined the effects of social support on psychological adjustment of newly diagnosed breast cancer patients. Because of increases in rates of incidence, prevalence, and survivorship of breast cancer, growing numbers of women are faced with the need to adapt to its diagnosis and treatments. Increased understanding of the role of social support in this adaptation process is of value to social workers involved with these patients.

REVIEW OF THE LITERATURE

Social Support and Illness

Studies have found that social support serves an ameliorating function during times of psychological distress in medical populations. Authors have proposed such a relationship in various populations including lung cancer patients (Quinn, Fontana, & Reznikoff, 1986), breast cancer patients (Ell, 1984; Funch & Mettlin, 1982; Hughes, 1982), and asthma and heart attack patients (Hammer, 1983). One explanatory model holds that the social network is a source of support in a crisis and thus a buffer against the harmful effects of stress (Hammer, 1983). Ell (1984) proposed that social relationships buffer individual perceptions of a stressor, provide resources to modify the environmental demand, and help manage individual affective response.

Social support has been positively associated with health status, but the specific pathways through which social support exerts its influence on health are not yet understood (Ell, 1984). Several sources have reported that social support may reduce the negative impact of stress on diverse health problems such as low birthweight, arthritis, and tuberculosis (Cobb, 1976; Hammer, 1983; Turner, 1981). Hammer postulated that the social network may be directly and causally involved in health outcomes, perhaps through the impact of social feedback on psychological processes. Social support is thought to help in reducing the amount of medication required, accelerating recovery, and facilitating compliance with prescribed medical regimens (Cobb, 1976). These effects may be due to an enhancement of self-esteem and sense of control, as well as an increased coping capacity, and may result in direct beneficial physical effects. Lipowski (1969) wrote, "the quality of the patient's interpersonal relationships at the time of onset of illness and during its course tend to have a profound effect on his experiencing illness and coping with it. The response of the family and other meaningful people to the patient's illness or disability, to his communications of distress, and to his inability to perform the usual social roles may spell the difference between optimal recovery or psychological invalidism." Lipowski cited three major sources of potential support: (1) physician or other medical personnel, (2) spouse and family, and (3) other patients.

Social Support and Cancer Patients

Social support and its effect on cancer patients' adjustment to diagnosis, treatment, and long-term survival have been studied extensively. Wortman (1984) and later Vernon and Jackson (1989) reviewed the literature in this area and summarized the fundamental constructs of social support as well as the findings and limitations of research available on this topic. Wortman pointed out that even though studies have found perceived support to be associated with positive outcomes, such as improved emotional adjustment or better coping, generally these studies have been correlational and have not provided evidence of a causal relationship between support and adjustment. Rather, social support has emerged as a predictor of adjustment (Wortman, 1984).

Although most of the empirical studies have focused on the effects of receiving support, some attention has also been given to factors that impede an individual's ability to mobilize and effectively use social support. Factors that deter support include prognosis, chronicity of illness, pain, type and location of symptoms, cultural and environmental influences, and characteristics of the provider (DiMatteo & Hays, 1981; House, 1981). Attention has also been given to the patient's psychological resources and the effect individual functioning has on the availability of social support as well as the effectiveness of this support in mitigating symptoms of distress and enhancing emotional adjustment (Schmale, 1984). Ell, Mantell, Hamovitch, and Niskomate (1989) used a multivariate approach to study the respective contributions of a sense of personal control and social support resources on the psychological outcomes of cancer patients. They concluded that personal control may be a more important coping mechanism than social support but that well-being is further enhanced by social resources.

Although most of the literature supports the belief that social support ameliorates stress, some empirical studies have not confirmed these findings. For example, Revenson, Wollman, and Felton (1983) found that supportive behaviors, defined as friendliness, understanding, useful information, and acts of tangible assistance, were not significantly related to measures of psychological adjustment.

Social Support and Breast Cancer

Meyerowitz (1980) evaluated the literature on psychosocial correlates of breast cancer and concluded that the emotional trauma that results from the diagnosis and treatment of cancer can be as potentially damaging as the disease itself, even for the most stable of women. In her study of breast cancer patients, Hughes (1982) found sustained emotional distress in 80 percent of subjects, of which 18 percent were found to be severely affected. Wolberg, Romsaas, Tanner, and Malec (1989) reported that psychological disturbances in patients diagnosed with breast cancer were found chiefly in assessments of mood and adjustment, the effects of which decreased over time but continued for at least

16 months postoperatively. Northouse and Swain (1987) found that at both three and 30 days postoperatively, breast cancer patients reported levels of psychological distress significantly above the level reported for the normal population. It is believed that depression, anxiety, and anger are widely experienced emotional reactions to the stress of facing cancer and its medical treatment (Meyerowitz, 1980).

Ell (1984) maintained that social support is an important predictor of coping with breast cancer. According to Meyerowitz (1980), certain aspects of the postdiagnostic environment can influence the degree of upset the patient feels in response to breast cancer, particularly the accessibility of emotionally supportive interpersonal relationships. Northouse (1988) reported that breast cancer patients with higher levels of support at both three and 30 days postoperatively had fewer adjustment problems than patients with lower levels of support. Likewise, Peters-Golden (1982) and Funch and Mettlin (1982) found that social support in breast cancer patients was positively related to psychological adjustment.

Ell (1984) cautioned, however, that relationships may also exert negative constraints or demands, one possible example being the husband of a breast cancer patient who is having difficulty with his own adaptation to the disease. Such a negative or nonsupportive dimension of social support was cited by Peters-Golden (1982). She suggested that negative support most often arises from a fear of death and dying or contamination of members of support networks and results in avoidance behaviors, which are in turn perceived by the breast cancer patient as a withdrawal of emotional support. Generally spousal support for breast cancer patients is positive and beneficial (Hughes, 1982; Quinn et al., 1986), the patient's husband being the most pivotal person in the support network (Peters-Golden, 1982).

Funch and Mettlin's (1982) findings confirmed the importance of support from spouse and family in helping breast cancer patients. Lichtman, Taylor, and Wood (1987) studied 78 breast cancer patients who were assessed an average of two years after surgery. They reported moderate correlations between perceived social support and psychological adjustment (r = .26 for family, .35 for friends, and .32 for husbands).

In contrast, Metzger, Rogers, and Bauman (1983) concluded that being married offered less of a protective buffer against the stress of breast cancer than expected. Another researcher who failed to find a relationship between support and well-being was Ehlke (1988), who studied physical symptom distress (defined as fatigue, insomnia, nausea, and pain) in 107 breast cancer patients receiving outpatient chemotherapy.

Defining Social Support

Although the term "social support" is widely used, general agreement as to the definition of this term is lacking. Previous studies have typically conceptualized social support in one of two ways, either from the perspective of social network size and function or from the perspective of perceived adequacy of support. Social network refers to the social connections provided by the environment in terms of structural (size, density, multiplicity) and functional (provision of information, comfort, emotional support, material aid) dimensions. Perceived social support refers to the impact networks have on the individual based on his or her subjective appraisal.

Studies using the concept of social support networks have demonstrated access only, which does not ensure that support is actually forthcoming or adequate (Ell, 1984). Procidano and Heller (1983) argued that differentiating perceived social support from the social network concept has value in that it is one step toward clarifying and operationalizing the social support variable. In addition, perceived adequacy of support has been found to be more predictive of positive outcome than availability of support (Ell, 1984).

Wortman (1984) identified five types of social support: (1) expression of positive affect or caring, (2) agreement with one's beliefs or feelings, (3) encouragement of open expression of beliefs and feelings, (4) provision of material aid, and (5) inclusion in a network of mutual or reciprocal help. Wortman reviewed the concept of social support as applied to cancer patients and suggested that social support assessments should look at both emotional support and tangible aid (for example, help with household chores, transportation, or child care). Wortman posited that different types of social support may be valuable to cancer patients at different points in their disease or treatment. Tangible support may be of greatest importance to the physically debilitated patient, whereas emotional support may be more valuable during early stages or remission.

The distinction between familial and nonfamilial sources of support is considered important, because different populations may rely on or benefit from these separate sources of support to different extents (Funch & Mettlin, 1982). In a 1985 study, Smith, Redman, Burns, and Sagert found that the marriage partner was the most important source of social support for married women who had been diagnosed one to three months before with reproductive cancers. For single women, relatives were found to provide the most support, with friends providing slightly less. In relation to the present study, it was of interest to consider how these different sources of social support contributed to patients' postdiagnostic psychological adjustment.

Although the concept of social support is widely used by social workers, careful scrutiny of the literature reveals multiple definitions for the term. This suggests that clinicians should consider the multi-faceted aspects of social support and carefully evaluate what types of support are needed by different groups of patients during different stages of illness. For example, the presence of family or friends to provide tangible assistance is critical for patients who are physically incapacitated by their disease. On the other hand, emotional support may be most valued by patients who have undergone disfiguring surgery, for example.

TABLE 1   Social Support Scores Reported by Married and Single Women, by Source of Support

Marital Status	Friend		Family		Spouse		Total	
	M	SD	M	SD	M	SD	M	SD
Single (n = 34)	31.9	6.1	27.9	8.9	NA	NA	67.8	12.6
Married (n = 101)	32.3	5.0	32.3	6.2	31.7	6.7	96.3	13.0
Total (n = 135)	32.2	5.2	31.2	7.2	25.8	11.9	89.1	17.9

NOTE: NA = not applicable.

METHOD

The present study addressed the effects of emotional support from three sources—family, friends, and spouses—as perceived and reported by breast cancer patients during the months immediately following active treatment of their cancer. Thus, both type of illness and stage of treatment were controlled, thereby allowing close examination of the relationship of degree and source of emotional support to psychological well-being.

Design

The original study, reported elsewhere, involved examining the impact of physician behavior during the cancer diagnostic interview on patients' subsequent psychological adjustment to breast cancer (Roberts, Cox, Reintgen, Baile, & Gibertini, in press). Social support, health status, and psychological adjustment before the cancer diagnosis were each measured to be included in the analysis as extraneous variables that were believed to play a significant role in patients' psychological well-being after treatment for breast cancer. Personality traits were assessed to determine if they influenced how the patient viewed her physician's behavior.

The present report provides an in-depth analysis of the degree and source of social support and their relationships to psychological well-being of breast cancer patients. Post hoc data analyses revealed important findings about the role of social desirability in respondents' descriptions of their social supports and in their self-reports of symptoms of psychological distress. Therefore, the social desirability variable was included in the design and data analysis.

Subjects

Recently diagnosed breast cancer patients treated at H. Lee Moffitt Cancer Center and Research Institute at the University of South Florida, Tampa, were invited to participate in the study. Eighty-five patients agreed to be a part of the study. An additional 50 patients treated at other facilities in Florida or

Illinois were recruited through professional meetings and newspaper announcements. This resulted in a total sample of 135 women, all of whom had breast cancer surgery between January 1989 and July 1990. Virtually all of the women were white and believed to be from the middle class, as reflected in the socioeconomic status of patients seeking care at this regional cancer center. The 50 subjects who responded to the newspaper advertisement were volunteers who expressed an interest in this type of research.

The average age of the patients was 56.2 years (SD = 11.9), with a range of 29 to 82 years. One hundred and one (75 percent) were married or in a spousal relationship, and 59 (44 percent) were employed outside of the home full- or part-time. Seventy-eight (58 percent) had a mastectomy, with the remainder choosing to have a lumpectomy, or surgical removal of the tumor and surrounding tissue, followed by radiation therapy. The research data collection was planned to take place approximately six months after breast cancer surgery. The actual time lapse averaged 5.8 months (SD = 2.1) for the sample.

Instruments

Degree and source of perceived social support were measured with a self-report instrument called the Social Support Questionnaire (SSQ) (Northouse, 1988). The SSQ was developed specifically to measure the quality of social support in breast cancer populations. The SSQ was derived from previous research on the support needs of mastectomy patients and included the following constructs: having a person who listens to concerns, demonstrates understanding, and shows love and concern, and having a person with whom the patient can discuss concerns and with whom the patient would not have to put on a false front (Northouse, 1988).

The SSQ asks subjects to rate the degree of support they perceived from three sources (spouse, family member, and friend) on each of eight items, yielding a total of 24 items within three subscales. Subjects rated each item (for example, "My spouse seems to understand what I am going through") on a five-point Likert scale ranging from 5 = strongly agree to 1 = strongly disagree. An overall total support score was calculated by summing the raw scores from each of the eight items on all three subscales, with higher scores indicating higher levels of support. A source of support score from each of the three subscales (spouse, family member, friend) was calculated by summing raw scores on the eight items within each subscale. Northouse (1988) reported reliability alpha coefficients of .90 on two separate administrations of the SSQ. The scale also showed evidence of concurrent validity.

Patients' current psychological status was assessed with the Standard Checklist-90-Revised (SCL-90-R), a standardized instrument that evaluates the psychological symptomatic distress of medical patients (Derogatis, 1983). It is a 90-item self-report symptom inventory assessing distress in nine dimensions—somatization, obsessive—compulsive behavior, interpersonal sensitivity, depression, anxiety, hostility, phobic anxiety, paranoid ideation, and psychoticism.

The Global Severity Index (GSI) constitutes the best single indicator of distress as measured by this instrument (Derogatis, 1983).

Social desirability was measured with the Desirability scale from the Personality Research Form—Form E (Jackson, 1984). People who score high on the Desirability scale describe themselves, either consciously or unconsciously, in favorable terms. According to Jackson, high scores may indicate conscious distortion to create a good impression. In other instances high scores may indicate the more subtle influences of very high self-regard or of being highly socialized and conforming. Jackson reported reliability coefficients ranging from .52 to .68 for the Desirability scale. Concurrent validity was found between the Desirability scale and the Achievement via Performance subscale of the California Psychological Inventory (r = .70).

Procedures

An introductory letter signed by the Breast Cancer Center's surgeons and the research social worker was sent to the patients to explain the study and request participation. Each patient then received a follow-up telephone call from the research social worker or a social work graduate student. Informed consent was obtained from women wishing to participate. The questionnaires were mailed to the subjects to complete and return.

Women solicited through newspaper announcements called the social workers to express their interest. Informed consent was obtained and questionnaires mailed approximately six months after surgery. Women who were married or in an ongoing relationship with a significant other were asked to complete all three subscales of the SSQ. The single women were asked to complete the family member and friend subscales.

RESULTS

The patients' level of psychological distress on the GSI was moderately elevated. The sample's average score represented a t score of 60 compared to a t score of 50 for the normative sample of nonpatient females (Derogatis, 1983). A t score of 60 represents one standard deviation above the mean. About 16 percent of nonpatient females would have this same or greater level of distress.

High levels of support from friends, family, and spouses were reported. The maximum score, indicating highest level of support, was 40 for each subscale. Patients who were married or living with a significant other could have scores that totaled 120, because they had three available sources of support, whereas single patients' maximum total support score was 80. The assumption that single women automatically have one-third less social support can be questioned, because these women may receive more attention from family

TABLE 2   Pearson Correlation Coefficients for Social Support and Psychological Distress, by Source of Support

Subsample	Family	Friend	Spouse	Total
Single women (n = 34)				
GSI	−.17	−.41(*)	NA	−.32
Depression	−.13	−.44(*)	NA	−.30
Anxiety	−.15	−.38(*)	NA	−.29
Married women (n = 101)				
GSI	−.12	−.01	−.27(**)	−.19
Depression	−.18	−.02	−.27(**)	−.22(*)
Anxiety	−.09	−.00	−.17	−.14
Total sample (n = 135)				
GSI	−.15	−.13	−.16	−.21(*)
Depression	−.18(*)	−.13	−.18(*)	−.23(**)
Anxiety	−.12	−.13	−.11	−.16

NOTE: GSI = Global Severity Index; NA = not applicable.
* p ≤ .05 . ** p ≤ .01.

members, particularly adult children, and may cultivate more relationships with friends. Therefore, all analyses were done for the entire sample, then broken down for married and single patients.

Table 2 contains the Pearson r's or product-moment correlation coefficients for the SSQ and the GSI. Correlations were also computed between the SSQ and the Depression and Anxiety subscales of the SCL-90-R. The rationale was that depression and anxiety experienced by breast cancer patients might more likely be ameliorated by social support than would other symptom dimensions.

Patients who scored high on the Desirability scale also reported high levels of support from spouses, friends, and family, with Pearson correlation coefficients ranging from .21 to .42. It was also observed that patients who scored high on desirability reported lower levels of psychological distress (r = −.43). Thus, it was decided to compute partial correlation coefficients that describe the relationship between two variables (social support and the GSI) while adjusting for the effects of a third variable, desirability. These partial correlations are shown in Table 3. Complete data were available for 125 subjects.

As can be seen in Table 3, when desirability is controlled, the correlations between social support and GSI scores drop to −.10 or less, with the exception of the −.18 correlation between spouse support and psychological distress of married women. When controlling for desirability, this correlation dropped in strength from −.27 to −.18, which reflects a weak but statistically significant relationship between higher spousal support and fewer symptoms of distress.

TABLE 3. Partial Correlation Coefficients for Social Support and Psychological Distress Controlling for Desirability

Subsample	Source of Support			
	Family	Friend	Spouse	Total
Single women (n = 30)	−.03	−.10	NA	−.02
Married women (n = 95)	−.07	−.01	−.18(*)	−.13
Total sample (n = 125)	−.03	−.05	−.01	−.03

NOTE: NA = not applicable.
p ≤ .05.

Perhaps the most dramatic change resulting from controlling for desirability scores is for single women who reported less distress in the face of good support from friends ($r = -.41$). After controlling for desirability, this correlation dropped to $-.10$.

DISCUSSION

On initial assessment of the data, a significant though modest relationship was found between perceived social support and psychological well-being of newly diagnosed breast cancer patients. The correlation coefficients were very similar to those reported by Lichtman et al. (1987), whose study used different measures of social support and of psychological symptoms. Additionally, the initial results supported the tentative hypothesis that single women with good support from friends received the same amount of psychological benefit that married women received from husbands' support.

The unanticipated finding that patients' social desirability scores were highly correlated with perceived social support and with self-report of psychological symptoms deserves careful scrutiny and further study. It appears that the influence of social desirability on cancer patients' responses and self-reports has not been addressed previously.

When the effect of social desirability was adjusted or controlled for, the correlations between social support and psychological distress were virtually eliminated, or in the case of spouses, substantially weakened. There are two possible interpretations regarding this finding. The first is that patients who wish to put the best face on their situation, consciously or unconsciously, are likely both to minimize their distress and to rate highly their spouses, families, and friends. Such patients may wish to convince themselves and others that they are handling this life crisis well and that they feel loved and cared for by their family and friends. This coping mechanism closely resembles denial, which has been shown to have value in ameliorating the stress encountered by cancer patients, particularly during certain stages of treatment (Wool & Goldberg, 1986).

A second interpretation follows from Jackson's (1984) second explanation of high scores on the Desirability subscale. He described high scorers as being highly socialized or possessing unusually high self-esteem. Following this line of reasoning, women high on social desirability may in fact cultivate more satisfying social relationships. Additionally, these women may have stronger coping mechanisms and good premorbid psychological adjustment that protects them from high levels of distress when diagnosed with breast cancer.

It is interesting that the social desirability factor had considerably less influence on the correlation of spouse support and psychological well-being of married women. It appears that spouse support has some stress–buffering value, though very modest, for breast cancer patients whereas support from other sources does not, and women may rate spousal support more realistically than other types of support. These interpretations are viewed as tentative but deserving of further study.

Wortman (1984) cautioned against interpreting correlations between social support and health outcomes as evidence for a causal relationship in which social support causes the outcomes. An alternative explanation for the relationship is that a poorly adjusted person is less likely to possess, establish, or benefit from a strong support system and less likely to adjust well to cancer. Results of this study underscore Wortman's point. In other words, the apparent correlation between support and adjustment may in fact lie within the person rather than within objective considerations of the support network.

This study raises the question of whether failure to assess personality or other person-centered variables in evaluating the relationship of social support to patient well-being may explain, in part, discrepant findings in previous research reported in the literature. For example, studies reporting a correlation between social support and adjustment may have used research subjects whose self-reports were influenced by the desirability factor.

Limitations of the Study

The social support literature discriminates between expressive or emotional support and tangible or material assistance. Further distinctions in measurements have been made between perceived support and social network size. Results from this study apply only to emotional support as perceived by the patients.

A second limitation stems from the sampling techniques, which were neither random nor stratified to ensure inclusion of women representing all races and socioeconomic classes. Thus, generalization of the findings can be made only to middle-class white women who agree to participate in studies of this type. The present subjects on average reported high levels of social support and likely had high levels of material support as well. A more representative sample might have resulted in greater variability in support and thus led to different conclusions.

Implications for Social Workers

Social workers trained in the person-in-situation configuration need to be particularly sensitive to this complex interaction in assessing the strength and helpfulness of patients' social support networks. The patient who describes a loving family and minimizes her distress may need a more in-depth assessment than initially appears; the data in this study indicate she is equally at risk to have psychological symptoms during the postdiagnostic phase. Conversely, the patient who acknowledges symptoms of depression and who is found to have a weak support system probably will need more intensive intervention than referral to a support group.

Multivariate analysis of predictors of psychological well-being were completed for the larger study and revealed that history of emotional problems and recent life stressors were more powerful predictors. Social workers should inquire first about past psychological adjustment and stressful life events in psychosocial assessments and accord social support a lesser role.

CONCLUSION

The results of this study affirm the conclusions of Revenson et al. (1983), who cautioned that social support is not the universal boon it is generally believed to be. Furthermore, the data lend considerable credence to previous speculations by authors such as Wortman (1984) that the characteristics of the person, rather than the situation, underlie the apparent relationship between social support and adjustment to illness.

REFERENCES

Cobb, S. (1976). Social support as a moderator of life stress. *Psychosomatic Medicine, 38,* 300–313.

Derogatis, L. R. (1983). *The SCL-90-R administration, scoring and procedures manual—II.* Towson, MD: Clinical Psychometric Research.

DiMatteo, M., & Hays, R. (1981). Social support and serious illness. In B. Gottlieb (Ed.), *Social networks and social support* (pp. 117–148). Beverly Hills, CA: Sage Publications.

Ehlke, G. (1988). Symptom distress in breast cancer patients receiving chemotherapy in the outpatient setting. *Oncology Nursing Forum, 15,* 343–346.

Ell, K. (1984). Social networks, social support, and health status. *Social Service Review, 58,* 133–145.

Ell, K., Mantell, J. E., Hamovitch, M. B., & Niskomate, R. H. (1989). Social support, sense of control and coping among patients with breast, lung and colorectal cancer. *Journal of Psychosocial Oncology, 7*(3), 63–89.

Funch, D. P., & Mettlin, C. (1982). The role of support in relation to recovery from breast surgery. *Social Science and Medicine, 16,* 91–98.

Hammer, M. (1983). Cored and "extended" social networks in relation to health and illness. *Social Science and Medicine, 17,* 404–411.

House, J. S. (1981). *Work, stress and social support.* Reading, MA: Addison-Wesley Press.

Hughes, J. (1982). Emotional reactions to a diagnosis and treatment of early breast cancer. *Journal of Psychosomatic Research, 36,* 277–283.

Jackson, D. N. (1984). *Personality Research Form manual.* Port Huron, MI: Research Psychologists Press.

Lichtman, R. R., Taylor, S. E., & Wood, J. V. (1987). Social support and marital adjustment after breast cancer. *Journal of Psychosocial Oncology, 5*(3), 47–74.

Lipowski, Z. J. (1969). Psychological aspects of disease. *Annals of Internal Medicine, 71,* 1197–1206.

Metzger, L. F., Rogers, T. F., & Bauman, L. J. (1983). Effects of age and marital status on emotional distress after a mastectomy. *Journal of Psychosocial Oncology, 1*(3), 17–33.

Meyerowitz, B. D. (1980). Psychosocial correlates of breast cancer and its treatments. *Psychological Bulletin, 87,* 108–131.

Northouse, L. L. (1988). Social support in patients' and husbands' adjustment to breast cancer. *Nursing Research, 37,* 91–95.

Northouse, L. L., & Swain, M. A. (1987). Adjustment of patients and husbands to the initial impact of breast cancer. *Nursing Research, 36,* 221–225.

Peters-Golden, H. (1982). Breast cancer: Varied perception of social support in the illness experience. *Social Science and Medicine, 16,* 483–491.

Procidano, M. E., & Heller, K. (1983). Measures of perceived social support from friends and family: Three validation studies. *American Journal of Community Psychology, 11,* 1–24.

Quinn, M. E., Fontana, A. F., & Reznikoff, M. (1986). Psychological distress in reaction to lung cancer as a function of spousal support and coping strategy. *Journal of Psychosocial Oncology, 4,* 79–90.

Revenson, T. A., Wollman, C. A., & Felton, B. J. (1983). Social supports as stress buffers for adult cancer patients. *Psychosomatic Medicine, 45,* 321–331.

Roberts, C. S., Cox, C. E., Reintgen, D., Baile, W. F., & Gilbertini, M. (in press). Influence of physician communication on newly diagnosed breast cancer patients' psychological adjustment and decision making. *Cancer.*

Schmale, A. H. (1984). Response to Camille Wortman. *Cancer, 53,* 2360–2362.

Smith, E. M., Redman, R., Burns, T. L., & Sagert, K. M. (1985). Perceptions of social support among patients with recently diagnosed breast, endometrial, and ovarian cancer. *Journal of Psychosocial Oncology, 3,* 65–81.

Turner, R. J. (1981). Social support as a contingency in psychological well-being. *Journal of Health and Social Behavior, 22,* 357–367.

Vernon, S. W., & Jackson, G. L. (1989). Social support, prognosis and adjustment to breast cancer. In K. S. Markides & C. L. Cooper (Eds.), *Aging, stress and health* (pp. 165–198). New York: John Wiley & Sons.

Wolberg, W. H, Romsaas, E. P., Tanner, M. A., & Malec, J. F., (1989). Psychosexual adaptation to breast cancer surgery. *Cancer, 63,* 1645–1655.

Wool, M. S., & Goldberg, R. J. (1986). Assessment of denial in cancer patients: Implications for intervention. *Journal of Psychosocial Oncology, 4,* 1–14.

Wortman, C. B. (1984). Social support and the cancer patient: Conceptual and methodological issues. *Cancer, 53,* 2339–2360.

DISCUSSION QUESTIONS

1. What is the purpose of this study? What were the authors interested in investigating?

2. What did the authors find?

3. What are the two possible interpretations that the authors suggest for their findings?

4. Comment on the fact that this was a correlational study. What does Wortman (1984) have to say about this issue?

5. What are the implications of this study for social workers treating women with breast cancer?

10

"If I Knew Then What I Know Now": Seropositive Individuals' Perceptions of Partner Trust, Safety and Risk Prior to HIV Infection

Tara L. Crowell and Tara M. Emmers-Sommer

ABSTRACT

The purpose of this study was to examine personal and relational characteristics of HIV positive individuals. Forty HIV positive heterosexuals, who were infected through heterosexual sex, completed an on-line questionnaire designed to assess perceived risk of HIV, perceived partner safety and trust, and reasons for these perceptions prior to HIV infection. Results indicated that prior to infection, HIV positive heterosexuals reported having similar sexual attitudes, beliefs, and behaviors to those not infected with the virus. Participants reported moderate to high levels of trust for their partners, low levels of perceived risk of infection, and high levels of perceived partner safety. A moderately

Communication Studies, Winter 2001 v52 i4 p302(22)
"'If I Knew Then What I Know Now': Seropositive Individuals' Perceptions of Partner Trust, Safety and Risk Prior to HIV Infection" by Tara L. Crowell and Tara M. Emmers-Sommer. © 2001 Central States Communication Association

strong, negative, linear relationship existed between perceived partner safety and partner trust and perceived risk. In addition,. women perceived their partners as "safer" than did men and those in serious relationships perceived their partners as safer than those in casual relationships. Results from this study shed light on the personal and relational characteristics of heterosexuals living with HIV and the utility of social comparison theory in raising awareness about HIV positive and negative individuals.

INTRODUCTION

Human immunodeficiency virus (HIV), the virus responsible for acquired immune deficiency syndrome (AIDS), was isolated and identified in 1981 (Gallo et al., 1984). Since the official identification of this virus, the number of reported cases of HIV and AIDS has grown rapidly in the United States and other countries (Ahituv, Hotz & Philipson, 1996). Subsequently, AIDS is now recognized as one of the most serious infectious disease epidemics of modern time. Despite the rapid rise in infection, the Centers for Disease Control (CDC) (2000) released a warning that people are continuing to engage in behaviors that put them at risk for sexually transmitted diseases. Because no current HIV vaccine or cure for AIDS exists, individuals must rely on personal factors to ensure safer sexual behaviors. Specifically, practicing safer sex involves a complicated process of believing in one's ability to engage in safer sex, as well as the interpersonal communication skills necessary to negotiate safer sex with a partner (Lear, 1995). Further, this willingness to engage in safer sexual communication may be the most important predictor of an individual's actual use (Adelman, 1991; Cantania, Coates, Stall, & Turner, 1992; Edgar, Hammond, & Freimuth, 1989; Lear, 1995; Oakley & Bogue, 1995).

According to the CDC (2001), as the millennium came to a close 21.8 million people had died from AIDS since the epidemic began, and 36.1 million people are estimated to be living with HIV/AIDS. Once perceived as a gay male disease, the demographics of the HIV/AIDS epidemic have changed. Fifty percent of new HIV infections occur in people under 25. In 1999, 1,813 young people (ages 13 to 24) were reported as living with AIDS, bringing the cumulative[1] total to 29,629 cases of AIDS in this age group (CDC, 2001). In the United States, HIV-related death has the greatest impact on young and middle-aged adults, particularly among racial and ethnic minorities. In 1998, HIV was the fifth leading cause of death for Americans between the ages of 25 and 44 (www.cdc.gov/hiv/pubs/facts/youth.htm). It has been estimated that at least half of all new HIV infections in the United States are among people under 25, and the majority of young people are infected sexually— 47% of all AIDS cases reported were acquired heterosexually. Women now account for 30% of new HIV infections, and as of 1999 most women (40%) reported with AIDS were infected through heterosexual exposure (www.cdc.gov/hiv/pubs/facts/women.htm). Similarly, the 1997 WHO report indicated that 75% of HIV infections in adults throughout the world were transmitted through unprotected sexual intercourse, and heterosexual intercourse (vaginal and anal) accounted for more than 70% of the cases. Further, many of these documented HIV/AIDS cases were a result of a single episode of heterosexual intercourse (Raghubir & Menon, 1998).

It is apparent that HIV is spreading rapidly among children, teenagers, heterosexual adult males and females, and senior citizens. Specifically, the CDC reported that out of the 36.1 million worldwide people living with HIV/AIDS, 16.4 million are women, and 1.4 million are children under 15. In 2000, the United Joint Nations Programme on HIV/AIDS (www.unaids.org) estimated that 920,000 adults and children in North America were living with HIV. Further, a recent press release revealed that 10% of the new HIV cases are individuals over the age of 50 (The National HIV/AIDS Conference Update, March 24, 1999). In short, the CDC stated that the overwhelming majority of people with HIV—approximately 95% of the global total—now live in the developing world (www.cdc.gov/hiv/stats/internat).

Even though heterosexual HIV cases continue to increase, individuals' perceived invulnerability still exists. Heterosexuals' misperception of risk of HIV may create a false sense of security that can result in risky sexual behavior. Past research indicates a positive relationship between perceived risk of HIV and condom use (e.g., Raghubir & Menon, 1998). Thus, individuals who have a greater perceived risk of HIV are more likely to engage in safer sexual behavior, including safer sexual communication. In support, recent research on HIV risk and social comparison theory (e.g., Rye, 1998) posits that if individuals view themselves as similar to someone who is HIV positive, they are more likely to engage in self-protection behaviors to reduce their risk of HIV. Indeed, a social comparison theoretical approach provides a strong framework from which to examine a possible link between HIV positive and negative individuals and how that link might be made through communicating experiences, attitudes and beliefs. Specifically, HIV negative individuals could learn from the experiences, attitudes, and beliefs held by HIV positive individuals prior to their infection, particularly if such experiences, attitudes, and beliefs compared similarly to their own. Such information could also inform health-related intervention techniques and educational programs.

Much of the personal relationships literature focuses on individuals who are HIV negative. Less research exists on those who are infected and the beliefs and behaviors held in their personal relationships that may have contributed to their seropositivity. Research needs to uncover whether current HIV positive individuals held beliefs and practiced certain communication behaviors that are similar to the profiles of current HIV negative individuals. If similarities do exist, becoming aware of them may provide a basis for effective future prevention methods. Given this, the purpose of this study is to investigate former levels of partner trust, perception of risk, and partner safety held by individuals currently living with HIV/AIDS who acquired the virus through heterosexual sex. Through the use of social comparison theory, the authors hope to uncover a profile of these individuals such that it informs HIV risk perceptions currently held by many HIV negative heterosexuals.

SOCIAL COMPARISON THEORY

Perceptions of invulnerability continue to influence individuals' sexual behavior and increase their level of risk. As Hooren and Buunk (1993) noted, it is impossible that the vast majority of a population will be better than average. In short, many individuals' perceived invulnerability is an illusion or an unrealistic perception, based on the statistical premise that the majority of the population cannot fall above the mean. From a social comparison theory perspective (Festinger, 1954), then, an individual's myth of invulnerability needs to be replaced with his/her actual levels of risk. HIV negative individuals may be able to realize what their actual level of risk is if they compare themselves to an HIV positive individual. If individuals perceive similarities between themselves and someone who is HIV positive, their differences become a less plausible rationale for their beliefs of invincibility. Past research argues that HIV negative individuals may be more likely to personalize the risk of AIDS if similarities between these two groups of individuals (HIV positive and HIV negative) are established (Fisher & Fisher, 1992; Fisher & Misovich, 1990). These findings suggest the power of homophily on perceptions of group membership; specifically, if HIV negative individuals perceive themselves as similar in attitudes and behaviors to HIV positive individuals, they might be more inclined to modify their attitudes and behaviors.

The potential influence of perceived similarities on behavior change has been explored through social comparison theory. Social comparison theory proposes that individuals evaluate their personal attributes and situations by comparing themselves with others (Buunk & Gibbons, 1997; Festinger, 1954; Suls & Wills, 1991), on a wide variety of dimensions: academic skills (Gibbons, Benbow, & Gerrad, 1994); attractiveness (Richins, 1991); current living situation (Bernstein & Crosby, 1980); coping abilities (Wood, Taylor, & Lichtman, 1985); health risk (Klein & Weinstein, 1998); illness symptoms (Sanders, 1982); and behavior cessation efforts (Gibbons, Gerrard, Lando, & McGovern, 1991). Further, past research suggests that social comparison processes may operate differently in non-threatening versus threatening situations (Tigges et al., 1998). For example, Wills (1981) proposed that when people are threatened, they tend to make downward comparisons; that is, they compare themselves with people who they see as different and worse off than themselves. Although social comparison theory has not been extensively applied to the study of risky sexual behavior, evidence for the existence of downward comparison has been documented in other health-related studies (for citations see Tigges, Wills, & Link, 1998, p. 862). For example, people coping with threats of spinal cord injuries, breast cancer, depression, smoking cessation, acutely ill newborns, and rheumatoid arthritis report engaging in downward comparisons. Downward comparisons with regard to HIV could be one explanation for why individuals evaluate their risk of infection as little or none.

Festinger (1954) believed that social comparison is often motivated by a desire for accurate self-evaluation. However, a substantial amount of more recent research shows that self-evaluation is but one of several reasons for people to engage in social comparison (e.g., Sun & Croyle, 1995). According to Wood (1989), social comparison serves at least three goals: self-evaluation, self-improvement, and self-enhancement/self-protection. First, Wood (1989) explained self-evaluation by stating "individuals strive to be accurate in their views of the world . . . so that they are accurate in self-evaluation" (pg. 232). Wood continued by explaining self-improvement as individuals' efforts to improve themselves; and self-enhancement/self-protection as individuals' behaviors/motives aimed at protecting or enhancing one's self-esteem. The social comparison literature argues that each of these goals is a possible motive behind social comparison.

Felson and Reed (1986) argued, "other people's performances and self-appraisals are sometimes highly predictive of our own self-appraisals" (p. 103). Further, the goal of self-enhancement or self-protection could provide the motivation an individual needs to personalize the risk of HIV and to engage in safer sexual communication and behavior (Fisher & Fisher, 1992a; Fisher & Fisher, 1992b; Fisher & Fisher, 1992c). In addition, researchers posited that when individuals judge their risk of negative outcomes, they might compare themselves with prototypes of individuals who experience these outcomes (Gibbon, Gerard & Boney McCoy, 1995; Klein, 1997; Weinstein, 1980).

One specific study that applies the principles of social comparison theory to increasing an individual's personalization of HIV reports promising results. Rye (1998) designed a study comprised of a treatment group and a control group. The treatment group was exposed to six HIV positive individuals that were defined as "people like us." The control group received no treatment. Statistical analyses comparing the two groups indicated that the individuals who received the treatment reported a significantly greater fear of HIV and a greater perceived risk of being infected with HIV than the control group. In addition, 56% of the individuals in the treatment group reported that they intended to use condoms in the future; 55% intended to talk to their partner about safer sex; and 28% reported that they would like to get an HIV test. Once individuals are able to personalize the risk of HIV, these beliefs are likely to act as a motivation for individuals to engage in safer sex communication and behavior.

The following section explores the research on safer sex attitudes. In particular, individuals' depersonalization of HIV risk is explored as influenced by their perceptions of risk, partner trust and partner safety.

DEPERSONALIZATION OF HIV RISK

Many individuals underestimate their level of risk by mentally drawing profiles of HIV positive individuals as very different from themselves. Research indicates that if individuals are unable to personalize the risk of HIV, they are unlikely to engage in safer sexual communication and/or behavior. However, personalization is more likely if an HIV negative individual knows someone who is HIV positive (or has died from AIDS), and has interpersonal contact with this person (Rye, 1998). Through interpersonal contact, individuals are more likely to connect with and relate to HIV positive individuals. Once the individual perceives similarities between him/herself and HIV positive individuals, he/she is much more likely to personalize the risk of AIDS. For example, during a focus group with six heterosexual HIV positive individuals, not one participant, prior to infection, believed he/she was similar to someone who was HIV positive (Crowell, 1999). More specifically, individuals within the focus group indicated that they did not use condoms because they perceived no need for them: "We were not the type of people who would get HIV." Overall, participants discussed their perceptions of invulnerability due to high partner trust and perceptions that their partner was "safe." Below, these constructs are discussed in further detail.

CONTRIBUTORS TO PERCEIVED INVULNERABILITY

Many factors may contribute to an individual's sense of invincibility. One attitude that interferes with an individual's adoption of safer sexual behaviors is feeling invulnerable to acquiring HIV (e.g., Ehde, Holm, & Robbins, 1995). Most heterosexuals continue to perceive that they are not at risk or are invulnerable, and therefore have not changed their behavior (e.g., Cantania et al., 1992). Wulfert and Wan (1995) argued that a major goal in developing more effective prevention and behavior change programs is to understand the psychological and social-psychological determinants of people's decisions to adopt or not to adopt AIDS risk reduction behaviors.

Partner Trust

Trust is one factor that may contribute to an individual's attitude of invulnerability. Researchers find that when partners indicate that they trust each other and believe they are in a monogamous dating relationship, they are less likely to use condoms than an individual who has multiple dating partners (Ishii-Kuntz, Whitbeck, & Simons, 1990). Crowell and Emmers-Sommer (2000) and Pilkington et al. (1994) found that participants who felt more positively about their partner and the relationship—trusted their partner, reported like/love and commitment for their partner—were less concerned about AIDS and STDs and were less influenced by these risks. Further, romantic feelings toward one's partner were associated with less fear of contracting AIDS and a lessened perceived susceptibility to contracting HIV. One possible explanation for these findings is that trust between couples increases as relationships grow, which leads to lower concern about contracting AIDS. For example, Metts and Fitzpatrick (1992) argued that condom use tends to be disregarded when partners achieve relational commitment and trust. Therefore, even if condoms are used in the early stages of a relationship, as the relationship progresses and trust is established, an individual's perceived need to use condoms for contraception often declines. If an individual believes his/her partner is faithful and not infected, they will likely perceive condom use as unnecessary. In addition, as the relationship progresses and trust increases, condoms may no longer be the primary or desired form of contraception, and alternate forms of birth control are often sought (Crowell & Emmers-Sommer, 2000; Lear, 1995; Maticka-Tyndale, 1991; Metts & Fitzpatrick, 1992; Sonnex, Hart, Williams, & Adler, 1989).

Among heterosexual couples, condoms are typically considered to be a method for birth control rather than a means for preventing sexually transmitted diseases (Maticka-Tyndale, 1991; Sonnex et al., 1989). As a result, if a couple uses another birth control method, such as the pill, they may be less inclined to use, or perceive a need to use a condom. "Sexually active [heterosexual] couples tend to use other forms of contraceptives (typically birth control pills), reducing the risk of pregnancy but increasing the risk of exposure to AIDS" (Metts & Fitzpatrick, 1992, p. 3).

Safe Partner

A second factor that contributes to an individual's attitude of invulnerability is the idea of a "safe partner." More specifically, an individual may perceive that there is no need to use condoms because his/her partner is "safe"; and he/she does not perceive him/herself as engaging in unsafe sex. Metts and Fitzpatrick (1992) stated:

> It is misleading however to assume that all people who engage in sexual intercourse without using condoms are unaware of or have flagrant disregard for safer-sex practices. Many sexually active people do not use condoms, but assume they engage in safer sex because they have intercourse only with persons they believe to be "safe." (p.1)

Thus, another determinant of an individual's decision regarding condom use is his/her perceived need for the use of condoms.

As stated earlier, individuals may perceive little, if any, need to use condoms because they believe they already engage in safer sex by choosing a partner who is "safe" (Metts & Fitzpatrick, 1992). One study indicated that the "most popular prophylactic" was the selection of a noninfected sexual partner (Ishii-Kuntz, Whitbeck, & Simons, 1990). Ishii-Kuntz et al. (1990) found that college students' confidence in the safety of their partner stemmed from two presumptions. First, an individual usually chooses a partner from within his/her own social network; and, therefore, the partner is presumed to be safe. In support, Timmins, Gallois, McCamish, and Terry (1996) found that an individual's perceived personal risk was influenced most by perceived risk of friends and of people with the same sexual practices. The second presumption is that "unsafe" people are somehow distinguishable from safe people, and can be recognized and avoided as sexual partners.

Two other predominant contributors to an individual's perception of a "safe" partner are: (1) a perception of a monogamous relationship, and (2) length and seriousness of the relationship (Crowell & Emmers-Sommer, 2000). Hence, an individual who believes he/she is in an exclusive relationship, has known the partner for a long time, or believes the relationship is serious reports little or no need for and use of condoms.

An individual's perception of invulnerability holds dangerous implications when coupled with research on extramarital affairs and cheating. Frank Pittman, author of *Private Lies: Infidelity and the Betrayal of Intimacy,* estimated that 60% of men and 40% of women have had or will have an extramarital affair (as cited in *USA Today,* February 10, 1998; Emling, 2000). Stebleton (1993) found that 36% of men and 21% of women at a Midwestern university reported being sexually unfaithful to his/her partner. Moreover, he found that 3/4 of men and 1/3 of women "never did ask" partners about past sexual history, and men admitted they lied to sexual partner(s) more often than women. Similarly, Cochran and Mays' (1990) results indicated that both men and women lie to their partners in order to obtain sex; specifically, "both men and women frequently reported that they would actively or passively deceive a dating partner in an effort to gain sex" (p. 777). Finally, a recent study indicated that four out of every ten HIV infected individuals (surveyed at two New England hospitals) failed to inform sex partners about their condition. Nearly two thirds of these individuals also reported they do not always use a condom (CNN News, 1998).

In order to ascertain the level of individuals' perceived invulnerability, partner trust, and perceived partner safety and the relationship between among these factors, the following research questions are posed to heterosexuals living with HIV:

RQ1: What was an individual's perceived risk of acquiring HIV prior to acquiring the virus?

RQ2: What was an individual's level of trust for their partner prior to acquiring the virus?

RQ3: Did an individual perceive their partner as "safe" prior to acquiring the virus?

RQ4: Does an individual's level of trust and perceived partner safety predict an individual's perceived level of risk?

RQ5: What reason(s) did an individual have for perceiving his/her level of risk of HIV infection, prior to obtaining the virus?

METHOD

Recruitment of Participants

Due to the specific criteria (i.e., HIV positive heterosexuals who obtained the virus through heterosexual, sexual contact) of the desired population, and the sensitive nature of the subject matter, collecting data on-line is one effective way to obtain this information. Recent studies found that an individual is more open with his/her responses when responding to questions on-line rather than when responding to paper and pencil surveys, especially with personal issues (CNN, 1998; Sell, 1997; Read, 1991). In addition, Sell (1997) posited that on-line surveys have the "ability to reach relatively rare, hidden, and geographically dispersed populations" (p. 297). One specific study conducted by IBM (Read, 1991), which 90% of their employees completed, reveals several advantages of on-line surveys over traditional paper and pencil surveys. Specifically, the study suggests the following benefits: (a) employees prefer it, (b) it is faster, (c) it is more flexible and easier to analyze, (d) it is more efficient, (e) employees give more open responses, and (f) employees provide more written comments (30 to 35% increase in responses to open-ended questions). Although on-line surveys are a relatively new method of data collection, they hold great promise in reaching numerous populations, especially those dealing with rare diseases, and/or specific health behaviors/interests (Sell, 1997). Therefore, for this study, an on-line questionnaire consisting of the various instruments outlined below was constructed in order to address the proposed research questions.

Participants were solicited from on-line news groups, AIDS hotlines and support groups, AIDS chat lines, and AIDS organization web pages. This process proved to be a substantial undertaking, extremely time-consuming, and difficult. The following provides a detailed description of the steps involved in soliciting participants.

First, a search of AIDS newsgroups was conducted on http://wren.supernews.com, and the results of this search yielded a list of newsgroups with a focus on HIV/AIDS. Every week for a two-month period, the first author posted a message to these newsgroups soliciting participants. Next, a comprehensive search of all Internet sites that deal with AIDS was performed. This task was accomplished by using dogpile.com, a search engine that scans all other search engines—GoTo.com, Yahoo, Thunderstone, Excite Guide Search, Excite Web Search, Minning Co., Lyco's Top 5%, Lyco's, Altavista, Info Seek, What U Seek; Web Crawler, and Magellan. First, the key words "AIDS" and "HIV" were searched. This search yielded over 5,000 relevant sites. Due to the extremely large number, the search was narrowed by using the key words "AIDS" and "support." This search produced approximately 500 sites.

The first author then read through the list of these sites and, based on the name and description, visited those that appeared to be possibilities for recruiting participants (organizations, groups, or individuals that appeared to have direct contact—face-to-face or communication via Internet or print—with HIV positive heterosexuals). After many hours of surveying these sites, it became apparent that there were three types of sites: (a) informative sites; (b) organizations for treatment and support sites; and, (c) personal and social sites. If sites were strictly informative—offered new information on HIV, treatment, prevention, medication, and contact information—the first author learned of other possible links from these pages, but did not use these sites for recruitment of participants (see Appendix B for examples of sites). The second type of web site, those of specific organizations across the United States, directly addressed individuals living with HIV. Information on these web sites indicated that these organizations have direct and daily access to individuals living with HIV. Thus, these web sites were used for the recruitment of possible participants.

Recruitment of possible participants from these organizations entailed a series of steps. First, the first author's recruitment message was sent to each web site that had an e-mail address for contacting a representative (90% of these sites have an e-mail address for a contact person). In addition, phone calls were made to each organization that listed a phone number. Phone calls contained roughly the same information as in the recruitment message. Many times the contact person at the organization would instruct the first author to put the request in writing and mail or fax him/her the request with a copy of the survey (between 15 to 20 letters were faxed or mailed). The letters followed the same format as the e-mail recruitment message—the first author's name, phone number, e-mail address, and affiliation, the purpose of the study, a description of potential participants, and, the web site address. Finally, flyers advertising the web site were sent to organizations that agreed to display the flyers in their office (see Appendix C for a list of all AIDS organizations that were either contacted by e-mail, phone, or both).

The third type of web site included was a personal web page of individuals living with HIV or organized chat rooms that offered support for individuals living with AIDS. Some of these web sites were categorized by sexual orientation; but most catered to all individuals living with AIDS, regardless of how the disease was transmitted or sexual preference. Personal web sites always contain an e-mail address to contact the person. There were approximately 10 to 12 personal homepages accessed using the same message posted on the organizations' web site. Web page owners at three of these sites linked the first author's survey site to their home pages. Two or three others sent e-mails to the first author indicating that they were not eligible to participate, but would relay the web site address to others. Some of these same individuals were also members of the chat groups and e-mailed the first author indicating that they would send a message about the study to the chat groups. Most of the chat groups were exclusive, meaning one needed to be HIV positive to even visit the site. Therefore, the first author was unable to post recruitment messages on those particular sites and, instead, sent direct e-mail messages to the web masters for these chat rooms and asked them to post a message in the chat room asking for assistance with the first author's on-line survey. About half the chat rooms posted the message, and the other half denied the request for a variety of reasons. The main reason was the sensitive nature of the questions; another reason was that the members felt that the purpose of the chat rooms was support, rather than solicitation (see Appendix D for a list of personal web pages and chat rooms contacted by the first author).

Sample

Participants in the study were 40 heterosexual individuals diagnosed with HIV. All individuals were infected with the virus through heterosexual sexual contact. The sample consisted of 16 males (40%) and 24 females (60%). The unequal distribution of gender in this sample appears representative of the population of HIV positive heterosexuals (those acquiring the virus through heterosexual contact), as women are 19% more likely to obtain HIV through heterosexual sexual activity than men (CDC, 1997).

Participants ranged in age from 21 to 55 with a mean age of 39.2 years. Thirty-three participants reported their race as white[2], while seven indicated that they were African American. In addition to these demographic variables, participants also provided information on relationship status and duration prior to infection, knowledge of their HIV infection, and birth control methods prior to infection.

With respect to relationship status and duration, four (10%) participants reported being single (not having sexual relations with anyone in particular), two (5%) reported causally dating someone, seven (17.5%) reported casually dating multiple partners, five (12.5%) reported exclusively dating one partner, three (7.5%) reported exclusively dating multiple partners, 13 (32.5%) reported cohabiting, five (12.5%) reported being married, and one (2.5%) reported being engaged. The length of these relationships was measured by the number of months that the partners were/are together. The length of relationships ranged from one month to 384 months (32 years), with an average of 72.5 months (approximately six years). Additionally, participants indicated who they acquired the virus from: five (12.5%) from a spouse, 12 (30%) from a boyfriend/girlfriend, four (10%) from someone they were causally dating, five (12.5%) from an acquaintance, two (5%) from a friend, two[3] (5%) from a fiance (fiancee), and two (5%) from an extra marital affair. Two (5%) participants did not know whom they obtained the virus from; and six (15%) participants did not provide this information.

Instruments

Perceived Risk.   Considering that this study is interested in individuals' perceived risk of acquiring HIV prior to actually obtaining it, participants were asked to respond to the five statements (adapted from Pilkington et al., 1994): 1) I was afraid of getting HIV; 2) I was not worried about getting AIDS; 3) There was high risk of being exposed to the HIV; 4) I was not the kind of person who was likely to get HIV; and 5) I was less likely than most people to get HIV. Participants responded to each of the five statements using the following scale: strongly agree = 1, agree = 2, unsure = 3, disagree = 4, strongly disagree = 5. Questions one and three were reverse coded to ensure reliability. The five-item perceived risk scale was subjected to a confirmatory factor analysis (CFA) using Hamilton and Hunter's (1988) CFA program. All five items loaded on one factor, ave $r = .72$, standard score alphas $= .93$.

Reliability of the overall scale was a very acceptable .93 (Cronbach's alpha) (see Table 1 for the correlation matrix, means, and standard deviations of risk items at www.infotrac-college.com). Respondents were also asked to provide a reason why they perceived this level of risk. Reasons for perception of risk were coded and categorized with coding methods used in similar studies (e.g., Crowell & Emmers-Sommer, 2000; Emmers & Canary, 1996). Specifically, reasons for risk perception were coded and then collapsed with similar other reasons to create overall themes. When a response did not correspond with other responses, a new category was formed. These categories were used to identify similar themes in the reasons why participants perceived a certain level of risk. Due to the small number of participants and the exploratory nature of this study, quantitative statistical analyses were not conducted with these data. Furthermore, the last statement that the participants responded to did not address a specific research question, and therefore intercoder reliability was not conducted.

Trust. Larzelere and Huston's (1980) The Dyadic Trust Scale, a unidimensional scale, was used to measure interpersonal trust in romantic relationships. Participants responded to each of the eight statements using the following scale: 1 = completely agree; 2 = strongly agree; 3 = agree; 4 = unsure; 5 = disagree; 6 = strongly disagree; 7 = completely disagree. The eight-item dyadic trust scale underwent a confirmatory factor analysis (CFA), using Hamilton and Hunter's (1988) CFA program. All eight items loaded on one factor, ave $r = .58$, standard score alphas $= .91$. Reliability of the overall scale was an acceptable .84 (Cronbach's alpha) (see Table 2 for the correlation matrix, means, and standard deviations of trust items at www.infotrac-college.com).

Perceived Safety of Partner. Although perceptions of a "safe" partner are often discussed in the literature, they are not often measured as a separate construct. Many times, the perception that a partner is "safe" falls under the larger umbrella of perceived invulnerability and is measured by level of risk of acquiring HIV. However, this construct is an individual's perceived level of risk due to perceptions of partner safety. Therefore, an individual's perception of partner safety was assessed independently from perceived risk. Participants' perception of partner safety was measured as follows: "Prior to obtaining HIV, how safe did you perceive the partner you obtained HIV from?" (Very Unsafe = 1, Unsafe = 2, Neutral = 3, Safe = 4, Very Safe = 5).

RESULTS

Research Question One asked, "What was an individual's perceived risk of acquiring HIV prior to acquiring HIV?" Results of the descriptive analyses reveal that participants' perceived risk ranged from 1 to 5 with a mean score of 2.57 and SD of 1.34, indicating a low level of perceived risk of obtaining HIV (see Table 3 for distribution of scores).

TABLE 3   Distribution or Perceived Risk Scores

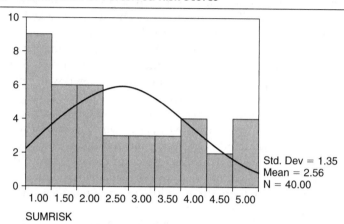

SUMRISK

Key: 1 = Strongly Agree; 2 = Agree; 3 = Unsure; 4 = Disagree; 5 = Strongly Disagree.

Research Question Two asked, "What was an individual's level of trust for their partner prior to acquiring HIV?" Results of the descriptive analyses reveal that participants' perceived trust for their partner ranged from 1.75 to 7 with a mean score of 4.36 and SD of 1.71, indicating a moderate level of perceived trust for partner (see Table 4 for distribution of scores).

TABLE 4   Distribution of Trust Scores

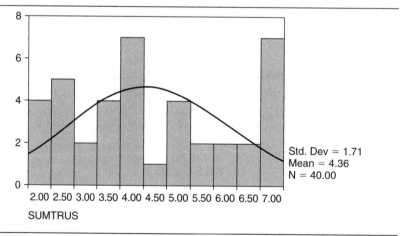

SUMTRUS

Key: 1 = Completely Agree; 2 = Strongly Agree; 3 = Agree; 4 = Unsure; 5 = Disagree; 6 = Strongly Disagree.

TABLE 5   Distribution of Safe Partner Scores

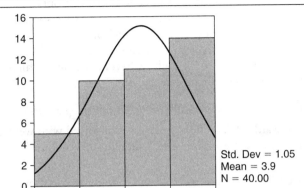

Key: 1 = Very unsafe; 2 = Unsafe; 3 = Neutral; 4 = Safe; 5 = Very Safe

Research Question Three asked whether or not individuals perceived their partner as "safe" prior to acquiring HIV. Results of the descriptive analyses reveal that participants' perceived partner safety ranged from 2 to 5 with a mean score of 3.85 and a SD of 1.05, indicating a moderately high perceived partner safety level (see Table 5 for distribution of scores).

Research Question Four asked whether or not an individual's level of trust and perceived partner safety would predict his/her perceived level of risk. Results of a multiple linear regression, with two predictors, reveal that both perceived trust of a partner and perceived partner safety were significant predictors of an individual's perceived risk ($F (2, 37) = 14.388$, $p < .001$), with slightly more than 40% of the variance in perceived risk explained by perceived partner trust and partner safety ($R^2 = .437$, adjusted $R^2 = .407$). Standardized coefficients reveal significant t values and negative betas for each predictor.

Beta t Sig.

Trust −.353 −2.720 .010

Partner Safety −.461 −3.553 .001

The t values indicate that each variable significantly accounts for the reduction in error when predicting an individual's perceived risk of HIV. In addition, the beta statistic identifies a negative relationship between perceived partner trust and perceived risk, and perceived partner safety and perceived risk. Thus, the less an individual trusted and perceived their partner as safe, the more risk he/she perceived of acquiring HIV. Prior to infection, then, participants in this study perceived high trust and safety in regard to their partner and thus perceived low risk of acquiring HIV.

Research Question Five asked, "What reason(s) did individuals state for perceiving their level of risk of HIV infection, prior to obtaining the virus?" Each participant's reason(s) were grouped with similar responses from other participants to form categories. When a participant's reason(s) did not correspond to an existing category, a new category was established. Participants' reason(s) were grouped to form eight different reasons, which were then collapsed into three supraordinate categories:

1. Sexual Behavior: "I was not gay" or "I did not sleep around"
2. Attitudes Toward HIV: "The women I was involved with were not sleazy" or "I was like everyone else, I thought it could never happen to me."
3. Relationship Status: "I was married and thought the relationship was exclusive" or "My partner told me he was HIV negative and I believed him."

The three reasons that referred to Sexual Behavior were reasons regarding sexual orientation, promiscuity, and drugs/alcohol. The reasons that referred to Attitude Toward HIV were reasons regarding perceived vulnerability and perceived safety of partner. The three reasons that referred to Relationship Status were reasons regarding trust for partner, monogamous relationships, and love for partner. Frequencies of the reported reasons indicate 31 sexual behavioral reasons for participants' perceived risk level, 21 reasons addressing participants' attitude toward HIV, and 19 reasons identifying participants' relational status (see Table 6 for the description and frequencies of the three supraordinate categories and the eight specific reasons at www.infotrac-college.com).

Additional Analyses

Although the research questions did not specifically ask for difference between males and females and perceived trust in partner, perceived HIV risk, and perceived safety of partner, or relational status and these same three dependent variables, t-tests were conducted to determine if any significant between-groups differences existed. Results reveal males (M = 3.06) and females (M = 4.37) significantly differed on perceived partner safety (t (38) = −4.864, p < .001); but did not differ on perceived risk of HIV (t(38) = .955, p > .05), or trust in partner (t(38) = −1.217, p > .05). T-tests were also conducted to assess the difference between relationship status and each of these three dependent variables. Relationship status was collapsed into two categories. Casual relational status was assigned to participants who indicated their status as either single (not seeing anyone in particular), casually dating one partner, or casually dating multiple partners. Serious relationship status was assigned to participants who indicated their status as either exclusively dating one partner, exclusively dating multiple partners, cohabiting with a partner, engaged, or married. Participants in casual relationships (M = 3.33) significantly differed from those in serious relationships (M = 4.16) in their perceptions of partner safety (t(38) = −2.576, p < .014); but they did not differ in their perceived risk of HIV (t(38) = 1.677, p > .05) or perceived trust in partner (t(38) = −1.410, p > .05).

DISCUSSION

Results of this study indicate that individuals living with HIV reported perceiving a low risk of being infected with HIV prior to infection. Perceived invulnerability with the current HIV positive sample is consistent with past findings revealing that invincibility is a major reason why HIV negative individuals engage in unprotected sexual activity (e.g., Ehde et al., 1995). The relationship between level of perceived risk and condom use is not a new revelation in the safer sex literature. However, determining that a low level of perceived risk was present for those who are now infected has significant implications for future prevention messages and methods. From a social comparison theory perspective, results from this study suggest that HIV positive individuals recall holding attitudes that are similar to those other researchers have found for HIV negative individuals (Crowell & Emmers-Sommer, 2000; Ishii-Kuntz et al., 1990; Metts & Fitzpatrick, 1992; Pilkington et al., 1994; Timmins et al., 1996).

Considering the notions of homophily and social comparison, implications can be drawn from the current study's findings to how HIV negative individuals might compare themselves to HIV positive individuals. Specifically, based on the premise of self-appraisal, if individuals compare themselves (i.e., perceive ourselves as similar) to prototypes of others who experience negative outcomes, these appraisals will be more predictive of their own self-appraisal (Felson & Reed, 1986). These appraisals might affect individual attitudes and subsequent behaviors. Similarly, relational partners could integrate safer sexual talk into their own relationships if they perceived themselves as similar in attitudes and behaviors as HIV positive couples due to their own appraisal. Recent research indicates that couples who integrated safer sexual talk into their relational script were more likely to engage in safer sexual behaviors (Allen, Emmers-Sommer, & Crowell, 2001). Future programs and prevention methods should take this information and use it advantageously.

In the past, research explored the relationships among trust, partner safety, and relationship status on HIV negative individuals' safer sex behaviors. In short, these studies indicated that each of these variables influenced an individual's safer sexual attitudes and behaviors (e.g., Raghubir & Menon, 1998). Specifically, the more individuals trusted their partners, the more likely they were to report a low perceived level of risk (e.g., Crowell & Emmers-Sommer, 2000; Lear, 1995). The same held true for partner safety (Ishii-Kuntz et al., 1990; Metts & Fitzpatrick, 1992). In the present study, participants' partner trust and perceived partner safety accounted for over 40% of the variance in individuals' perceived level of risk. In addition to trust and partner safety, relational status also impacted individuals' perceived level of risk. These findings support past research on long-term committed relationships or marital relationships in which partners often perceive little or no risk of contracting HIV due to their relational status (e.g., Emmers-Sommer & Crowell, 1999; Willing, 1994). In summary, the more an individual trusted his/her partner, and perceived him/her as "safe," and the longer and more committed the relationship, the less the individual believed he/she was susceptible to HIV. This relationship appeared with both HIV positive individuals in this study and in past research on HIV negative heterosexuals.

Partner trust significantly varied by relationship status. Individuals living with HIV who were in serious relationships perceived their partner as significantly safer than those in casual relationships. This relationship between perceived partner safety and relational status has also been identified in the heterosexual HIV negative population. Research on HIV negative heterosexuals indicates that individuals who believe they are in an exclusive relationship or have known their partner for a long time report little or no condom use. The findings of the current study correspond to the findings of past literature, in which individuals report that the safest sex is with a "safe" partner (Ishii-Kuntz et al., 1990; Metts & Fitzpatrick, 1992) and that unprotected sex relates to perceived monogamy and partner trust (Ishii-Kuntz et al., 1990).

Another similarity in perceived risk between HIV positive (prior to infection) and HIV negative individuals is the reasons individuals provide to explain perceived level of risk. Specifically, participants indicated that their sexual orientation, use of drugs, and promiscuity directly influenced their perceived level of risk. If individuals were heterosexual, did not use drugs, and were not promiscuous, they believed that they were at a low level of risk of infection. Finally, participants provided reasons associated with the status of their relationship. Examples include responses such as: (a) "I trusted my partner, he told me he was HIV negative and I believed him," (b) "We were monogamous," (c) "I was married and thought the relationship was exclusive," and (d) "Because he seemed to be in love with me."

The influence of attitudes of invulnerability on safer sex behavior has serious consequences when coupled with the potential unfaithfulness of partners. Individuals need to be aware that their partner may be putting them at risk even when they believe that they are in a "monogamous" relationship. Twenty-five participants (65%) in this study reported being in serious relationships prior to be infected. Further, 19 out of the 32 participants who indicated that they knew from whom they contracted the virus reported that they were in a serious relationship with that person (e.g., husband/wife, boyfriend/girlfriend, or fiance/fiancee).

Individuals in more committed relationships (i.e., serious dating, cohabiting, engaged, or married) perceive themselves as having a more stable and honest relationship than those who are in casual relationships (i.e., casual dating, romantic friends, or acquaintances) (Knapp, 1984). Yet, statistics suggest a high incidence of relational infidelity (e.g., Emling, 2000). Thus, a false sense of security may exist for individuals in serious relationship due to the contradiction between their perception of the relationship and the actual status of the relationship.

These findings hold dangerous implications for individuals, especially for women, who determine their level of risk based on trust, relational status, and partner safety. Results of this study revealed that women significantly differed from men on their perception of partner safety. Specifically, women reported perceiving their male partner to be safer than males perceived their female partner. Potentially dangerous consequences exist for women who inaccurately perceive their partner safety, particularly when considering that women are 19 times more likely to become infected from an HIV positive male (due to the exchange in bodily fluids between a man and a women), than a male is from an HIV positive female (CDC, 1998).

Delineating HIV positive heterosexuals' safer sex attitudes prior to infection helps researchers to better comprehend the personal and relational factors involved in transmission and possible ways to curb this transmission. Results of this study suggest that HIV positive heterosexuals, prior to infection, held many of the same attitudes about their level of risk as non-infected heterosexuals currently hold. These findings hold promise for the utility of social comparison theory in explaining similarities between HIV positive and negative groups and possible future behavior change. For example, Wood (1989) found that when individuals seek out social confirmation they choose the information that is readily available. Thus, availability of this type of information—actual attitudes, communication, and behavior of seropositive individuals—would prove fruitful to the awareness, understanding, and education of others.

This contention supports past research indicating individuals who have direct contact with seropositive individuals report less perceived invincibility. Klein (1997) argued that individuals seek out social confirmation of their own beliefs and behavior. Thus, if individuals are seeking out social confirmation on safer sexual attitudes and behavior, the accuracy for which they base these comparisons should be available. Once the realities of seropositive individuals are communicated to others, seronegative individuals might be more likely to engage in self-improvement and self-protection. In addition, future research should focus on similarities and differences among seropositive individuals. As with all groups, there are many demographic and psychographic characteristics that differ and influence members within a group. To maximize the theoretical potential for social comparison theory in increasing individuals' personalization of HIV, similarities and homophily will need to be apparent. Once highlighted, social comparison theory could raise individuals' awareness and decrease their level of invincibility; everyone potentially holds some level of risk.

LIMITATIONS

As with all research, this research is not without several limitations. First, the underrepresentation of a population in this study leads to limited generalizability of results. The researchers used a convenience sample and participants self-selected to the study based on their sexual orientation and mode of acquiring the virus. Thus, the results need to be interpreted with caution. In addition, the use of an n size of 40 was powerful enough to detect larger effect size in the statistical analyses; however, it was not large enough to reveal existing medium or small effects. A larger sample size would provide more depth and breadth in responses to the open-ended questions. Nevertheless, given the population of focus and existing literature on seropositivity, a sample size of 40 was deemed acceptable.

A second limitation of this study is that although it is comparative in nature, it is not a true comparison study (two groups). This study obtained results for one group to make comparisons, based on past research, to another group. One could argue that to determine true similarities between these two populations, both samples should have been represented in this study. However, the design of this study acted as a first step in the comparison process because it provides the descriptive and inferential information necessary about heterosexuals living with HIV in order to design a future study to determine the effectiveness of social comparison theory as means to personalization. Nevertheless, the researchers identified valuable similarities between the results of this study and those of past studies that collected data on HIV negative heterosexuals (primarily college students).

A third limitation relates to the actual data collection procedures. Collecting data on-line limited not only the number of individuals who could participate, but also the type of individuals. The majority of the participants were white adults, with only one minority group (African American) represented (although underrepresented). Statistics from the CDC (1998) illustrates that minorities are one of the fastest growing HIV positive populations, and therefore should be represented in HIV/AIDS research. The underrepresentation of minorities in past and present research around the world is an important issue that needs to be addressed in future endeavors. In addition, the possibility of obtaining an adequate representation of the HIV positive heterosexual population was hindered due to the exclusion of minorities' from higher economic and educational opportunities (i.e., factors affecting computer and online access, etc.).

As indicated above, this sample is not completely representative of the HIV positive heterosexual population. Therefore, future research should build upon this study through the use of improved methods data collection to obtain a more representative sample. Despite the drawbacks associated with sample representation of this study, the results offer significant, valuable information that contributes to our understanding of heterosexuals living with HIV.

NOTES

1.   Among both males and females in this age group, the proportion of cases with exposure risk not reported or identified (25% for males and 41% for females) will decrease and the proportion of cases attributed to sexual contact and injection drug use will increase as follow-up investigations are completed and cases are reclassified into these categories.

2.   The U.S. Census Bureau defines "White (not of Hispanic origin)" as "a person having origins in any of the original peoples of Europe, North Africa, or the Middle East."

3.   Only one person indicated that they were engaged at the time, but two people indicated that they obtained HIV from their fiance. Engaged was not one of the provided options for relational stages. The one participant wrote in the response "engaged" while the other may have chosen "exclusively dating one partner" or "living together."

REFERENCES

Adelman, M. B. (1991). Play and incongruity: Framing safe sex talk. *Health Communication, 3,* 139–155.

Ahituv, A., Hotz, V.J., & Philipson, T. (1996). The responsiveness of the demands for the local prevalence of AIDS. *Journal of Human Resources, 31,* 4, 869–898.

Allen, M., Emmers-Sommer, T. M., & Crowell, T. L. (2001). Negotiating safe sexual behavior. In M. Allen, R. Preiss, B. Gayle, & N. Burrell (Eds.), *Interpersonal communication: Advances in meta-analysis* (pp. 345–366). Hillsdale, NJ: Lawrence Erlbaum Associates.

Bernstein, M., & Crosby, F. (1980). An empirical examination of relative deprivation theory. *Journal Experimental Social Psychology, 16,* 442–456.

Buunk, B. P., & Gibson, F. X. (1997). *Health, coping, and well-being: Perspectives from social comparison theory.* Hillsdale, NJ: Lawrence Erlbaum Associates.

Cantania, J. A., Coates, T.J., Stall, R., & Turner, H. (1992). Prevalence of AIDS-related risk factors and condom use in the United States. *Science, 258,* 1101–1106.

Centers for Disease Control (1994). *HIV/AIDS surveillance report* (Vol. 6, No. 1).

Centers for Disease Control (1995). *HIV/AIDS surveillance report* (Vol. 7, No. 1).

Centers for Disease Control (1997). *Youth risk behavior surveillance* (Vol. 47, No. SS-3)

CNN Interactive (September 25, 1998). Teens prefer "telling all" to computers. Available HTTP: http:cnn.com/TECH/science/9805/14/t_t/teen.survey.technique/index.html [September 25, 1998]

CNN Interactive (February, 8, 1998). Study: Many people with AIDS virus don't tell sex partner. Available HTTP: http:cnn.com/HEALTH/9802/08/sexualethics.ap/[February 8, 1998].

Cochran, S. D., & Mays, V. M. (1990). Sex, lies, and HIV. *The New England Journal of Medicine, 1332,* 774–775.

Crowell, T. (1999). Investigating heterosexuals living with HIV: A focus group of a HIV positive heterosexuals' support group. Unpublished manuscript.

Crowell, T. L. & Emmers-Sommer, T. M. (2000). Examining self-efficacy, communicative coping styles, and reasons for condom nonuse in heterosexual relationships. *Communication Research Reports, 17* (2), 191–202.

Decarlo, P. (1996). What are Women's HIV prevention Needs? Available HTTP: http://www.epibiostat.ucsf, edu/capsweb/womentext.html [February 17, 1998].

Edgar, T., Freimuth, V. S., Hammond, S. L., McDonald, D. A., & Fink, E. L. (1992). Strategic sexual communication: Condom use and resistance and response. *Health Communication Research, 4,* 83–104.

Emling, S. (January 16, 2000). Cheating hearts make good business. Available HTTP: http://www.usatoday.com/life/ldso26.htm [January 17, 2000].

Emmers, T. M., & Canary, D.J. (1996). The effect of uncertainty reducing strategies on young couples' relational repair and intimacy. *Communication Quarterly, 44,* 166–182.

Emmers-Sommer, T. M., & Crowell, T. L. (1999). *The effect of reasons for condom use suggestion on certainty, trust, and intimacy in marital relationships.* Paper presented at the International Communication Association Convention, San Francisco, CA.

Ehde, D. M., Holm, J. E., & Robbins, G. M. (1995). The impact of Magic Johnson's HIV serostatus disclosure on unmarried college students' HIV knowledge, attitudes, risk perception, and sexual behavior. *Journal of American College Health, 44* (2), 55–58.

Felson, R. B., & Reed, M. D. (1986). Reference groups and self-appraisals of academic ability and performance. *Social Psychology Quarterly, 43,* 103–109.

Festinger, L. (1954). A theory of social comparison processes. *Human Relations, 7,* 117–140.

Fisher, J. D., & Fisher, W. A. (1992a). A general social psychological model for changing AIDS risk behaviour. In J. Pryor & G. Reeder (Eds.), *The social psychology of HIV injection* (pp. 127–253). Hillsdale, NJ: Lawrence Erlbaum Associates.

Fisher, J. D., & Fisher, W. A. (1992b). Changing AIDS risk. *Psychological Bulletin, 111,* 455–474.

Fisher, J. D., & Fisher, W. A. (1992c). Understanding and promoting AIDS preventive behaviour: A conceptual model and educational tools. *Canadian Journal of Human Sexuality, 1,* 99–106.

Fisher, J. D., & Misovich, D.J. (1990). Evolution of college students' AIDS related behavioral responses, attitudes, knowledge, and fear. *AIDS Education and Prevention, 2,* 322–337.

Gallo, R. C., Salahuddin, S. Z., Popovic, M., Shearer, G. M., Kaplan, M., Haynes, B.F., Palker, T.J., Redfield, R., Oleske, J., Safai, B., Whiter, F., Foster, P., & Markham, P. D. (1984). Human T-lymphortropic retrovirus, HTLV-III, isolated from AIDS patients and donors at risk for AIDS. *Science, 224,* 500–503.

Gibson, F. X., Benhow, C. P. & Gerrard, M. (1994). From top dog to bottom half: Social comparison strategies in response to poor performance. *Journal of Personality and Social Psychology, 67,* 638–652.

Gibson, F. X., Gerrard, M., & Boney McCoy, S. (1995). Prototype perception predicts (lack of) pregnancy prevention. *Personality and Social Psychology Bulletin, 21,* 85–93.

Gibson, F. X., Gerrard, M., Lando, H. A., & McGovern, P. G. (1991). Social comparison and smoking cessation: The role of the "typical smoker." *Journal of Experimental Social Psychology, 27,* 239–258.

Hamilton, M., & Hunter, J. (1988). *Confirmatory Factor Analysis.* Unpublished computer program, Department of Psychology, Michigan State University, East Lansing.

Hoorens, V., & Buunk, B. P. (1993). Social comparison of health risks: Locus of control, the person-positivity bias, and unrealistic optimism. *Journal of Applied Social Psychology, 23,* 291–302.

Ishii-Kuntz, M., Whitbeck, I. B., & Simons, R. I. (1990). AIDS and perceived change in sexual practice: An analysis of a college student sample from California and Iowa. *Journal of Applied Social Psychology, 20,* 1301–1321.

Klein, W. M. (1997). Objective standards are not enough: Affective, self-evaluations, and behavioral responses to social comparison information. *Journal of Personality and Social Psychology, 72,* 763–774.

Klein, W. M., & Weinstein, N. D. (1998). Social comparison and unrealistic optimism about personal risk. In B. P. Buunk & F. X. Gibson (Eds.), *Health, coping, and well-being: Perspectives from social comparison theory* (pp. 25–61). Hillsdale, NJ: Lawrence Erlbaum Associates.

Knapp, M. L. (1984). *Interpersonal communication and human relationships.* Boston, MA: Allyn & Bacon.

Kolata, G. (1989, October 8). AIDS is spreading in teenagers, a new trend alarming to experts, *New York Times,* pp. 1, 30.

Larzelere, R. E., & Huston, T. L. (1980). The dyadic trust scale: Toward understanding interpersonal trust in close relationships. *Journal of Marriage and the Family, 42*(3) 595–603.

Lear, D. (1995). Sexual communication in the age of AIDS: The construction of risk and trust among young adults. *Social Science Medicine, 41,* 1311–1323.

Maticka-Tyndale, E. (1991). Sexual scripts and AIDS prevention: Variation in adherence to safer-sex guidelines by heterosexual adolescents. *Journal of Sex Research, 28,* 45–66.

Melts, S., & Fitzpatrick, M. A. (1992). Thinking about safer sex: The risky business of "knowing your partner" advice. In T. Edgar, M. A. Fitzpatrick, & V. S. Freimuth (Eds.), *AIDS: A communication perspective* (pp. 1–19). Hillsdale, NJ: Lawrence Erlbaum Associates.

Oakley, D., & Bogue, E. (1995). Quality of condom use as reported by female clients of a family planning clinic. *The American Journal of Public Health, 85,* 1526–1531.

Pilkington, C. J., Kern, W., & Indest, D. (1994). Is safer sex necessary with a "safe" partner? Condom use and romantic feelings. *The Journal of Sex Research, 31,* 203–210.

Raghubir, P., & Menon, G. (1998). AIDS and me, never the twain shall meet: The effects of information accessibility on judgments of risk and advertising effectiveness. *Journal of Consumer Research, 25,* 52–63.

Read, W.H. (1991, January). Gathering opinion on-line. *HR Magazine,* 51–53.

Richins, M. L. (1991). Social comparison and the idealized images of advertising. *Journal of Consumer Research, 18,* 71–83.

Rye, B. J. (1998). Impact of an AIDS prevention video on AIDS-related perceptions. *The Canadian Journal of Human Sexuality, 7,* 19–30.

Sanders, G. S. (1982). Social comparison and perceptions of health and illness. In G. S. Sanders & J. Suls (Eds.), *Social psychology of health and illness* (pp. 129–157). Hillsdale, NJ: Lawrence Erlbaum Associates.

Sell, R. L. (1997). Research and the Internet: An e-mail survey of sexual orientation. *American Journal of Public Health, 87,* 297.

Sonnex, C., Hart, G. J., Williams, P., & Adler, M.W. (1989). Condom use by heterosexuals attending a department of GUM: Attitudes and behavior in the lights of HIV infection. *Genitourinary Medicine, 65,* 248–251.

Stebleton, M. J., & Rothenberger, J. H. (1993). Truth or consequences: Dishonest in dating & HIV/AIDS-related issues in a college age population. *Journal American College Health, 42* (5), 51–54.

Stevens, J. (1996). *Applied multivariate statistics for the social sciences* (3rd edition). Mahwah, NJ: Lawrence Erlbaum Associates.

Suls, J., & Wills, T. A. (1991). *Social comparison: Contemporary theory and research.* Hillsdale, NJ: Lawrence Erlbaum Associates.

Sun, Y., & Croyle, R. T. (1995). Level of health threat as a moderator of social comparison preferences. *Journal of Applied Social Psychology, 25*, 1937–1952.

Tigges, B. B., Wills, T. A., & Link, B. G. (1998). Social comparison, the threat of AIDS, and adolescent condom use. *Journal of Applied Social Psychology, 28*, 861–887.

Timmins, P., Gallois, C., McCamish, M., & Terry, D. (1996). *Sources of information about HIV/AIDS and perceived risk of infection among heterosexual young adults: 1989 and 1994.* Paper presented at the 46th Annual Conference of the International Communication Association, Chicago, Ill.

USA Today (February 10, 1998). Liaisons test the bond of marriage. http://www.usatoday.com/life/health/sexualit/1hsex001/htm [February 10, 1998].

Weinstein, N. D. (1980). Unrealistic optimism about future life events. *Journal of Personality and Social Psychology, 39*, 803–820.

Wills, T. A. (1981). Downward comparison principles in social psychology. *Psychological Bulletin, 90*, 245–271.

Willing, C. (1994). Marital discourse and condom use. In P. Aggleton, P. Davie, & G. Hart, AIDS: *Foundations for the future* (pp. 110–121). London, England Taylor and Francis.

Wood, J. V. (1989). Theory and research concerning social comparison of personal attributes. *Psychological Bulletin, 106*, 231–248.

Wood, J. V., Taylor, S. E., & Lichtman, R. R. (1985). Social comparison in adjustment to breast cancer. *Journal of Personality and Social Psychology, 49*, 116–1183.

Wulfert, E., & Wan, C. K. (1995). Safer sex intentions and condom use viewed from a health belief, reasoned action, and social cognitive perspective. *The Journal of Sex Research, 32*, 299–311.

DISCUSSION QUESTIONS

1. The authors use a social comparison model to approach their research questions. Why do they think this is a useful approach to understanding perceived risk of contracting HIV? Comment on the role of similarity in their model.

2. What is the purpose of this study?

3. What did the authors find? What was people's level of perceived risk of contracting HIV prior to getting the disease? How much did people trust their partner prior to contracting HIV?

4. What are the implications of these findings for people in committed relationships who do not practice safe sex all of the time?

5. Describe one of the limitations of this study.

11

Risk Factors for Intimate Partner Violence and Associated Injury among Urban Women

Benita J. Walton-Moss, Jennifer Manganello, Victoria Frye, and Jacquelyn C. Campbell

ABSTRACT

The objective of this study was to identify risk factors for abuse and IPV related injury among an urban population. This study reports an additional analysis of a case-control study conducted from 1994 to 2000 in 11 USA metropolitan cities where of 4746 women, 3637 (76.6%) agreed to participate. Control group women (N = 845) were identified through random digit dialing. Significant risk factors for abuse included women's young age (adjusted odds ratio (AOR) 2.05 p = .011), being in fair or poor mental health (AOR 2.65 p < .001), and former partner (AOR 3.33 p < .001). Risk factors for partners perpetrating IPV included not being a high school graduate (AOR 2.06 p = .014), being in fair or poor mental health (AOR 6.61 p < .001), having a problem with drug (AOR 1.94 p = .020) or alcohol use (AOR 2.77 p = .001), or pet abuse (AOR 7.59 p = .011). College completion was observed to be protective (AOR 0.60, p < .001). Significant risk factors for injury included partner's fair or poor mental health (AOR 2.13, p = .008), suicidality (AOR 2.11, p = .020), controlling behavior (AOR 4.31, p < .001), prior domestic violence arrest

Journal of Community Health, Oct 2005 v30 i5 p377(13)
"Risk Factors for Intimate Partner Violence and Associated Injury Among Urban Women" by Benita J. Walton-Moss, Jennifer Manganello, Victoria Frye, and Jacquelyn C. Campbell. © 2005 Plenum Publishing Corporation

(AOR 2.66, p = .004), and relationship with victim of more than 1 year (AOR 2.30, p = .026). Through integration of partner related risk factors into routine and/or targeted screening protocols, we may identify more abused women and those at greater risk of abuse and injury.

INTRODUCTION

Intimate partner violence (IPV) is a major cause of morbidity and mortality for women in the United States (US). According to the National Violence Against Women Survey (NVAWS) approximately 25.5% of US women reported IPV (physical or sexual assault) or stalking at least once in their lifetime. (1) Past year IPV prevalence in population-based surveys has ranged from 1.5% to 13.6%. (1,2) According to estimates from the National Crime Victimization Survey (NCVS), 20% of the violent crime committed against women between 1993 and 2001 was attributed to IPV and at least one-third of female homicide victims were killed by an intimate partner. (3) IPV is currently the most common cause of nonfatal injury in the US. (4) Between 1992 and 1996, 36% of emergency department visits made by women were related to IPV. (5) Our definition of intimate partner violence is taken from a consensus panel for the U.S. Centers for Disease Control and Prevention (CDC) as follows: physical and/or sexual assault or threats of assault against a married, cohabitating, or dating current or estranged intimate partner by the other partner, also including emotional abuse and controlling behaviors in a relationship where there has been physical and/or sexual assault. (6)

Identifying abused women is increasingly being acknowledged as a potential way to decrease the morbidity and mortality associated with IPV. Thus, identifying risk factors for IPV is an important public health endeavor. In population and clinic based samples, the following factors differentiated physically abused from non-abused women: educational achievement discordance, (7) specifically when the woman has a higher education than her partner, cohabitating, (2) unmarried, (2,7) African American, (2) young age, (7) low income without health insurance or Medicaid, (7) cigarette use, history of physical abuse, self perceptions of poor physical and mental health (8) and children in the home. (8)

Thompson et al. (8) sought to identify factors associated with injury of a woman due to abuse by her partner by comparing risk factors for IPV in two national surveys, the Canadian Violence Against Women Survey (CVAWS) and the NVAWS. Results indicated that children witnessing partner violence, partner's alcohol use, history of prior victimization by the same partner and the woman reporting fear of injury or death were associated with physical injury. However, only two factors, partner's alcohol use and chronic victimization by the same partner, were independently associated with injury in both data sets.

As an increasing number of professional association guidelines and health care agencies and facilities implement targeted and universal IPV screening or routine inquiry, (9,10) it is helpful to be able to offer empirically validated profiles of women likely to suffer abuse, and the partners likely to perpetrate it. It is particularly important that such results emanate from population-based surveys as they are more likely to be generalizable to the population of women in the US. Identifying risk factors for abuse and injury resulting from abuse is critical for designing interventions to prevent, screen, and treat IPV. Thus, the objective of this analysis is to identify risk factors for IPV and IPV related injury among an urban random sample of women who were the control group of a case control study of intimate partner homicide.

METHODS

Setting and Participants

The case control study of intimate partner homicide was conducted in 11 geographically dispersed US cities from 1994 to 2000. (11) Cases were women who had survived an attempted homicide (n = 183) or proxies of women who did not (typically mothers, sisters, or friends) (n = 220). A control group was also included to compare with the cases. Women in the control group were identified through random stratified digit dialing from the same metropolitan areas as the femicide cases. A total of 4746 women met the age (18–50) and relationship criteria (intimate partner within the past year) and were read the full consent statement as approved by the Johns Hopkins University Institutional Review Board (IRB) as well as a local IRB at each site. Of these, 3637 (76.6%) agreed to participate. A modified version of the Conflict Tactics Scale (12) was used to identify abused women. Women who reported physical and/or sexual assault or being threatened with a weapon during a current or past relationship within the past 2 years constituted the abused group (n = 427). An equal number of nonabused women comprised the control group (n = 418), randomly selected from women who reported no abuse during the past 2 years.

Assessments

All controls interviewed included questions on sociodemographic factors, relationship characteristics, weapon availability, drug use, psychological abuse, perceived mental health of self and partner and prior arrest of partner, as well as responses to standardized instruments such as the Danger Assessment (13) and the HARASS. (14) Additionally, the same five questions used in the CVAWS (8) to evaluate emotional abuse were used in this study. A safety protocol was implemented, adopted from the telephone safety domestic violence protocol developed by Holly Johnson that includes providing domestic violence resources for all participants. (15) This analysis is a comparison of the abused with the nonabused women in the control group.

Statistical Analysis

Data were analyzed with STATA, version 8. (16) Univariate and bivariate analyses were conducted to determine differences between abused and nonabused women including t–tests for continuous variables and Chi–square tests for categorical variables. Backward stepwise logistic regression analysis was then utilized for those variables noted to be statistically significant at the $p \leq$ level in the bivariate analyses for inclusion in the multivariate model. Missing data (~9%) was handled by substituting mean or median values as appropriate. This was not done for the injury analysis.

RESULTS

The prevalence of intimate partner violence in the sample was 9.8% (n = 356). Most of the women in the sample were over 25 years of age (as were their partners), unmarried, living without children in the home, a high school graduate, and employed full time. Approximately half (53%) of the sample was White, 19% African American, 19% Hispanic, and 8% of "other" ethnic background. The association of abuse status and woman-level, partner-level, and relationship-level characteristics hypothesized to be related to IPV from prior research were investigated through bivariate analysis. All of the woman-level characteristics, and all but one of the partner-level characteristics were significantly associated with abuse. The only partner-level characteristic not associated with abuse was history of ever being in the military. Similarly, the only relationship-level characteristic not associated with abuse was the presence of a biological child of the woman but not the partner's (stepchild) in the home. Table 1 illustrates the findings of the bivariate analyses.

In the multivariate analysis, two characteristics of the women were independently associated with abuse: younger age and fair or poor mental health. Women who were less than 26 years of age were about twice as likely to be abused. Women who reported fair or poor mental health were more than twice as likely to be abused compared with the non-abused group. In contrast, five partner characteristics were associated with abuse, including not being a high school graduate (adjusted odds ratio (AOR) 2.05), woman's perception that the partner's mental health was fair or poor (AOR 6.61), woman's perception of partner's problem drug (AOR 1.94) or "Did he ever follow you or spy on you?" Finally, 7.42% of the nonabused women answered "yes" to no more than 1 question for the emotional abuse CVAWS questions, for example, "He calls you names to put you down or make you feel bad." There were however, particular items from these scales that differentiated injured women from non-injured physically abused controls. Injured women were much more likely to report that their partner made unwanted calls (40% vs. 2%, p < .0001), restricted them from talking with others (63% vs. 3%, p < .0001),

TABLE 1   Associations by Abuse Group

	Abuse	
	N (%) Total	(n = 427) n (%)
Woman's Characteristics n = 845		
Age		
18–25 years	219 (25.92)	154 (36.07)
26–50 years	626 (74.08)	273 (63.93)
Employment		
Full time (reference)	494 (58.6)	233 (54.57)
Part time	147 (17.44)	89 (2.84)
No job	204 (24.14)	105 (24.59)
Education		
Not high school graduate	101 (12.01)	70 (16.51)
High school graduate	740 (87.99)	354 (83.49)
Race/Ethnicity		
Black	161 (19.24)	96 (22.80)
White (reference)	447 (53.41)	200 (47.51)
Hispanic	160 (19.12)	92 (21.85)
Other	69 (8.24)	33 (7.84)
Individual Income		
≤ $20,000	416 (49.23)	254 (59.48)
>$20,000	429 (50.77)	173 (40.52)
Health		
Excellent/Good	730 (86.39)	345 (80.80)
Fair/Poor	115 (13.61)	82 (19.20)
Mental Health		
Excellent/Good	674 (79.76)	288 (67.45)
Fair/Poor	171 (20.24)	139 (32.55)
Problem Drinker	37 (4.38)	30 (7.03)
Drug Use	85 (10.08)	57 (13.38)
Partner's Characteristics		
Age		
18–25 years	180 (21.3)	135 (31.62)
26–50 years	665 (78.7)	292 (68.38)
Employment		
Full time (reference)	661 (79.16)	284 (67.78)
Part time	79 (9.46)	52 (12.41)
No job	105 (12.43)	91 (21.31)
Education		
Not high school graduate	146 (17.85)	108 (26.47)
High school graduate	672 (82.15)	300 (73.53)
College graduate	326 (38.58)	109 (33.54)

Continued

TABLE 1 *Continued*

	Abuse	
	N (%) Total	(n = 427) n (%)
Race/Ethnicity		
Black	185 (32.08)	108 (25.47)
White (reference)	440 (52.51)	192 (45.28)
Hispanic	158 (18.85)	93 (21.93)
Other	55 (6.56)	31 (7.31)
Health		
Excellent/Good	719 (85.09)	330 (77.28)
Fair/Poor	126 (14.91)	97 (22.72)
Mental Health		
Excellent/Good	597 (70.65)	210 (49.18)
Fair/Poor	248 (29.35)	217 (50.82)
Problem Drinker	159 (18.84)	133 (31.15)
Drug Use	157 (18.6)	130 (30.44)
Partner ever in military	127 (15.17)	69 (16.35)
Partner ever arrested for violence outside home	55 (6.7)	46 (11.27)
Partner ever had nonviolent arrest	13 (13.76)	84 (20.59)
Gun in home	141 (16.69)	68 (15.93)
Relationship Characteristics		
Relationship Status		
Current Partner	578 (68.4)	220 (51.52)
Former Partner	267 (31.6)	207 (48.48)
Relationship Status: Type		
Husband	340 (40.52)	107 (25.30)
Ex-Husband	34 (4.05)	32 (7.57)
Boyfriend	217 (225.86)	98 (23.17)
Ex-Boyfriend	132 (15.73)	104 (24.59)
Common law husband	3 (0.36)	2 (0.47)
Ex-Common law husband	5 (0.60)	4 (0.95)
Same-sex partner	12 (1.43)	10 (2.36)
Former Same-sex partner	0	0
Estranged husband★	9 (1.07)	8 (1.89)
Other	87 (10.37)	58 (13.71)
Biological Children in Home	268 (31.79)	112 (26.23)
Stepchildren in Home	138 (16.35)	78 (18.27)

TABLE 1   *Continued*

	Non-abused (n = 418)	
	n (%)	p value
Woman's Characteristics n = 845		
Age		<.001
18–25 years	65 (15.55)	
26–50 years	353 (84.45)	
Employment		.017
Full time (reference)	261 (62.74)	
Part time	58 (13.94)	
No job	99 (23.68)	
Education		<.001
Not high school graduate	31 (7.43)	
High school graduate	386 (92.57)	
Race/Ethnicity		.002
Black	65 (15.63)	
White (reference)	247 (59.38)	
Hispanic	68 (16.35)	
Other	36 (8.65)	
Individual Income		<.001
≤$20,000	162 (38.76)	
>$20,000	256 (61.24)	
Health		<.001
Excellent/Good	385 (92.11)	
Fair/Poor	33 (7.89)	
Mental Health		<.001
Excellent/Good	386 (92.34)	
Fair/Poor	32 (7.66)	
Problem Drinker	7 (1.67)	<.001
Drug Use	28 (6.71)	.001
Partner's Characteristics		
Age		<.001
18–25 years	45 (10.77)	
26–50 years	373 (89.23)	
Employment		<.001
Full time (reference)	377 (90.63)	
Part time	27 (6.49)	
No job	14 (3.35)	
Education		<.001
Not high school graduate	38 (9.27)	
High school graduate	372 (90.73)	
College graduate	217 (66.56)	

Continued

TABLE 1 *Continued*

	Non-abused (n = 418)	
	n (%)	p value
Race/Ethnicity		<.001
Black	77 (18.6)	
White (reference)	248 (59.9)	
Hispanic	65 (15.7)	
Other	24 (5.8)	
Health		<.001
Excellent/Good	389 (93.06)	
Fair/Poor	29 (6.94)	
Mental Health		<.001
Excellent/Good	387 (92.58)	
Fair/Poor	31 (7.42)	
Problem Drinker	26 (6.24)	<.001
Drug Use	27 (6.46)	<.001
Partner ever in military	58 (13.98)	.338
Partner ever arrested for violence outside home	9 (2.18)	<.001
Partner ever had nonviolent arrest	29 (7.02)	<.001
Gun in home	73 (17.46)	.549
Relationship Characteristics		
Relationship Status		<.001
Current Partner	358 (85.65)	
Former Partner	60 (14.35)	
Relationship Status: Type		<.001
Husband	233 (56.01)	
Ex-Husband	2 (.48)	
Boyfriend	119 (28.36)	
Ex-Boyfriend	28 (6.73)	
Common law husband	1 (0.24)	
Ex-Common law husband	1 (0.24)	
Same-sex partner	2 (0.48)	
Former Same-sex partner	0	
Estranged husband*	1 (0.24)	
Other	29 (6.40)	
Biological Children in Home	156 (37.50)	<0.001
Stepchildren in Home	60 (14.39)	0.128

* (still married, no legal action).

TABLE 2 Crude and Adjusted ORs for Predictors of Abuse

Characteristics	Crude OR (95% CI)	Adjusted OR (95% CI)
Woman's Characteristics (n = 845)		
Age		
18–25	3.06 (2.20, 4.26)	2.05 (1.18, 3.57)
26–50	1.0 (Referent)	1.0 (Referent)
Mental health		
Fair/poor	5.82 (3.85, 8.80)	2.65 (1.59, 4.49)
Good/excellent	1.0 (Referent)	1.0 (Referent)
Partner's characteristics		
Education		
<High school	3.52 (2.36, 5.26)	2.06 (1.16, 3.66)
≥ High school	1.0 (Referent)	1.0 (Referent)
College graduate	0.32 (0.24, 0.43)	0.60 (0.37, 0.95)
Not college graduate	1.0 (Referent)	
Mental health		
Fair/poor	12.9 (2.20, 4.26)	6.61 (4.00, 10.43)
Good/excellent	1.0 (Referent)	1.0 (Referent)
Alcohol		
Problem drinker	6.8 (2.20, 4.26)	2.77 (1.60, 4.78)
Not problem drinker	1.0 (Referent)	1.0 (Referent)
Drug use		
Problem w/drugs	6.59 (2.20, 4.26)	1.94 (1.11, 3.39)
No problem	1.0 (Referent)	
Pets		
Pet abuse	19.15 (2.20, 4.26)	7.59 (1.61, 35.96)
Relationship characteristics		
Former partner	5.61 (2.20, 4.26)	3.33 (2.02, 5.49)
Current partner	1.0 (Referent)	1.0 (Referent)

Characteristics	p-value
Woman's Characteristics	
Age	
18–25	.011
26–50	
Mental health	
Fair/poor	<.001
Good/excellent	

Continued

TABLE 2 *Continued*

Characteristics	p-value
Partner's characteristics	
Education	
<High school	.014
≥ High school	
College graduate	<.001
Not college graduate	
Mental health	
Fair/poor	<.001
Good/excellent	
Alcohol	
Problem drinker	.001
Not problem drinker	
Drug use	
Problem w/drugs	.020
No problem	
Pets	
Pet abuse	.011
Relationship characteristics	
Former partner	<.001
Current partner	

wanted to know everything (74% vs. 7%, p < .0001), and called the victim names (33% vs. 3%, p < .0001), as compared with non–injured physically abused women.

DISCUSSION

We found in this study that young women, reporting fair or poor mental health, or women separated from their partners, were more likely to be abused. Perpetrators of IPV were more likely to have not graduated from high school, have problems with drug or alcohol use, be in fair or poor mental health, and have a history of threatened or actual pet abuse. Women whose partners completed college were significantly less likely to be abused. These findings generally concur with those from the NVAWS (1) and the Behavioral Risk Factor Surveillance System (BRFSS), (7) and many other population-based and clinical studies. (2,17,18) In particular, there was overlap with our findings with respect to the following factors: relatively young age, separated or divorced marital status, substance use, and perceptions of poor mental health. As has been pointed out in other studies, since this is cross-sectional data, we do not know if the separation or divorce that is associated with IPV came before the violence or occurred after or both. Similarly, it could be that abused women were more likely to leave their partners, not that ex-partners were more likely to abuse women.

Although our findings of association of pet abuse with IPV has been observed in other investigations, (19–21) ours is the first controlled investigation that we have found. This risk factor is particularly important as Flynn (20) as well as Faver and Strand (21) observed that for some abused women, concern for their pet's welfare delayed their seeking shelter and safety from their abusers. This factor has also been incorporated in some clinical settings as exemplified by Siegel and colleagues who reported use of a brief screen for domestic violence in the pediatric setting that included a question inquiring about pet abuse. (22)

In addition, we found no independent associations between abuse status and presence of a stepchild in the home, as has been found by Daly, Singh and Wilson. (23) It is important to note that the presence of stepchildren in the home was significantly associated with intimate partner femicide in the larger case-control study from which these data come (11) as was also found by Daly, Wiseman, and Wilson. (24) We also found no independent associations between abuse and race or ethnicity; consistent with findings from the NVAWS (1) and other population-based studies in the US (25–27) as well as the larger parent study when risk of intimate partner femicide was the outcome. (11)

We also found that women whose partners had a prior domestic violence arrest, was in a relationship with their partner for more than 1 year, and who perceived their partner to be controlling, in fair or poor mental health, or suicidal were more likely to be injured compared to physically abused women who were not injured. In our study partner's alcohol problem was not independently associated with injury status unlike the CVAWS (8) and NVAWS. (1) In these studies women were asked about their partner's use of alcohol at the time of abuse and while we also asked women about partner's alcohol use when they were injured in our study, we also asked about their perceptions of their partner's lifetime problematic alcohol use.

In this study, the self-rated mental health of both the woman and her partner were consistently related to abuse and injury status. It is unclear, however, whether mental health status is not a precursor of abuse and/or injury, or if it instead reflects an outcome of being abused and injured. Women's perceptions of poor mental health however, may be a useful marker for case finding. Although some women may not initially disclose their abuse status, they are frequently well-known to the health care system for a myriad of physical and mental health problems known to be associated with abuse. (28) Through careful listening health care providers may suspect abuse based on references she makes about her or her partner's mental health. (29)

The finding that the presence of a gun in the home increased the risk of injury by more than three times for women underscores the danger of guns in cases of domestic violence. (11) Stalking behaviors were also associated with injury demonstrating the importance of assessment for stalking in cases of domestic violence and to consider stalking as a form of IPV. (30–33)

This analysis importantly adds to the body of knowledge from population based studies of the prevalence and risk factors of IPV for women using a population based sampling approach. However, there are also important limitations. One limitation is that all partner-level characteristics were ascertained retrospectively and reported by the woman, not the male partner. However, other studies of abused women, such as both NVAWS (1) and CVAWS (8), have also relied on female partner self-reports on their male partners' characteristics and behaviors. Further, it is not well known what impact partner non-participation has on prevalence of risk factors or abuse. (34) The findings are also limited to urban women which increased the ethnic diversity of the sample but neglected an important segment of the population, rural women, about which little is known in terms of IPV. Since the questionnaire was designed primarily around risk factors for homicide and near homicide of abused women, important risk factors for IPV were not measured such as history of childhood abuse.

Nonetheless, the findings reported here have implications for current abuse screening practice in health care and social service settings. Among the woman characteristics, perceived mental health had the strongest relationship to abuse along with a similar strength of association to that of being separated from their abusive partner. Routine assessment for IPV should not be limited to women asserting current involvement in a relationship, particularly if they report poor mental health. Our findings that it is characteristics of the partner more so than the victim that are most strongly and most often associated with abuse reinforces the importance of focusing not primarily on the woman or her relationship, but on her partner's characteristics as risk factors for abuse in terms of both identification and intervention. Focusing on the partner accomplishes two things: (1) it more accurately identifies women who are being abused, and (2) it communicates that it is her partner who for the most part is in control of and responsible for the abuse, not her. By integrating partner-level characteristics into routine and/or targeted assessment protocols, we may identify more abused women and women at greater risk of abuse and injury.

Benita J. Walton-Moss, DNS, APRN, BC is Assistant Professor of Nursing; Jacquelyn C. Campbell, PhD, RN, FAAN is Professor of Nursing, both at Johns Hopkins University, Baltimore, Maryland; Jennifer Manganello, PhD, MPH is Assistant Professor at the Annenberg School for Communication, University of Pennsylvania, Philadelphia, Pennsylvania; Victoria Frye, DrPH is Investigator at the Center for Urban Epidemiologic Studies, New York Academy of Medicine, New York, NY, USA

Requests for reprints should be addressed to: Benita Walton-Moss, DNS, APRN, BC, School of Nursing, Johns Hopkins University, 525 North Wolfe Street, Baltimore, Maryland 21205, USA; e-mail: bmoss@son.jhmi.edu.

REFERENCES

1. Tjaden PJ, Thoennes N. *Full Report of the Prevalence, Incidence, and Consequences of Violence Against Women: Findings from the National Violence Against Women Survey.* Washington, D.C.: National Institute of Justice, 2000NCJ-183781.

2. Jones AS, Gielen AC, Campbell JC, Schollenberger J, Dienemann JA, Kub J, O'Campo P, Wynne EC. Annual and lifetime prevalence of partner abuse in a sample of female HMO enrollees. *Women's Heath Issues* 1999; 9:295–305.

3. Rennison CM. *Intimate partner violence, 1993–2001.* Bureau of Justice Statistics Crime Data Brief. February 2003, NCJ 197838. http://www.ojp.usdoj.gov/bjs. Accessed 9–12–03.

4. Kyriacou DN, Anglin D, Taliaferro E, et al. Risk factors for injury to women from domestic violence against women. *N Engl J Med* 1999; 341:1892–1896.

5. Rand MR. *Violence-related injuries treated in hospital emergency departments.* Bureau of Justice statistics, Special Report. Washington, DC: US Department of Justice, August 1997.

6. Saltzmann LE, Fanslow JL, McMahon PM, Shelley GA. *Intimate Partner Violence Surveillance: Uniform Definitions and Recommended Data Elements, Version 1.0.* Atlanta, GA: National Center for Injury Prevention and Control, Centers for Disease Prevention, 1999.

7. Vest JR, Catlin TK, Chen JJ, Brownson RC. Multistate analysis of factors associated with intimate partner violence. *Am J Prev Med* 2002; 22:156–164.

8. Thompson MP, Saltzman LE, Johnson H. A comparison of risk factors for intimate partner violence-related injury across two national surveys on violence against women. *Violence Against Women* 2003; 9:438–457.

9. The Commonwealth Fund. Health Concerns across a Woman's Lifespan. *The Commonwealth Fund 1998 Survey of Women's Health.* New York: Commonwealth Fund, 1999.

10. The Commonwealth Fund. *Domestic Violence Prevention Evaluation Report.* New York: Commonwealth fund, 2004.

11. Campbell JC, Webster D, Koziol-McLain J, Block C, Campbell D, Curry MA, Gary F, Glass N, McFarlane J, Sachs C, Sharps P, Ulrich Y, Wilt SA, Manganello J, Xu X, Schollenberger J, Frye V, Laughon K. Risk factors for femicide in abusive relationships: Results from a multi-site case control study. *Am J Public Health* 2003; 93:1089–1097.

12. Straus MA. Measuring intrafamily conflict and violence: The conflict tactics scales. *Journal of Marriage and the Family* 1979; 41:75–88.

13. Campbell JC, Webster D, Koziol-McLain J, Block CR, Campbell DW, Curry MA, Gary FA, McFarlane J, Sachs C, Sharps PW, Ulrich Y, Wilt SA. Assessing risk factors for intimate partner homicide. *NIJ Journal* 2003; 250:14–19.

14. Campbell J, McKenna L, Torres S, Sheridan D, Landenburger K. Nursing care of survivors of intimate partner violence. In JC Humphreys and JC Campbell (Eds.). *Family Violence in Nursing Practice.* Philadelphia: Lippincott, Williams & Wilkins, 2003.

15. Johnson H, Sacco VF. Researching violence against women: Statistics Canada's national survey. *Canadian Journal of Criminology* 1995; 37:281–304.

16. *STATA Version 8.0.* Stata Corporation 2003.

17. Dearwater SR, Cohen JH, Campbell JC, Nah G, Glass N, McLoughlin E, Bekemeir E. Prevalence of intimate partner abuse in women treated in community emergency health departments. *JAMA* 1998; 280:433–438.

18. Harris RM, Sharps PW, Allen K, Anderson EH, Soeken K, Rohatas A. The interrelationship between violence, HIV/AIDS, and drug use in incarcerated women. *J Assoc Nurses AIDS Care* 2003; 14:27–40.

19. Ascione FR. Battered women's reports of their partners' and children's cruelty to animals. *J Emotional Abuse* 1998; 1:119–133.

20. Flynn CP. Woman's best friend. Pet abuse and the role of companion animals in the lives of battered women. *Violence Against Women* 2000; 6:162–177.

21. Faver CA, Strand EB. To leave or to stay? Battered women's concern for vulnerable pets. *J Interpersonal Violence* 2003; 18:1367–1377.

22. Siegel RM, Joseph EC, Routh SA, Mendel SG, Jones E, Ramesh RB, Hill TD. Screening for domestic violence in the pediatric office: a multipractice experience. *Clin Pediatr* 2003; 42:599–602.

23. Daly M, Singh LS, Wilson M. Children fathered by previous partners: A risk factor for violence against women. *Canadian J of Public Health* 1993; 84:209–210.

24. Daly M, Wiseman KA, Wilson M. Women and children sired by previous partners incur excess risk of uxoricide. *Homicide Studies* 1997; 1:61–71.

25. Schafer J, Caetano R, Clark C. Rates of intimate partner violence in the United States. *Am J of Public Health* 1998; 88:1702–1704.

26. Bauer HM, Rodriguez MA, Perez-Stable EJ. Prevalence and determinants of intimate partner abuse among public hospital primary care patients. *J Gen Intern Med* 2000; 15:811–817.

27. Rennison C, Planty M. Nonlethal intimate partner violence: examining race, gender, and income patterns. *Violence and Victims* 2003; 18:433–442.

28. Campbell JC. Health consequences of intimate partner violence. *Lancet* 2002; 359:1331–1336.

29. Sharps PW, Koziol-McLain J, Campbell J, McFarlane J, Sachs C, Xu X. Healthcare providers's missed opportunities for preventing femicide. *Prev Med* 2001; 33:373–380.

30. Burgess AW, Harner H, Baker T, Hartman CR, Lole C. Batterers' stalking patterns. *Journal of Family Violence* 2001; 16:309–322.

31. Logan T, Leukefeld C, Walker B. Stalking as a variant of intimate violence: implications from a young adult sample. *Violence and Victims* 2000; 15:91–111.

32. McFarlane J, Campbell JC, Watson K. Intimate partner stalking and femicide: urgent implications for women's safety. *Behav. Sci. Law* 2002; 20:51–68.

33. Mechanic M. The impact of severe stalking experienced by acutely battered women: an examination of violence, psychological symptoms and strategic responding. *Violence and Victims* 2001; 15:443–458.

34. Waltermaurer EM, Ortega CA, McNutt L. Issues in estimating the prevalence of intimate partner violence. *Journal of Interpersonal Violence* 2003; 18:959–974.

DISCUSSION QUESTIONS

1. Comment on the severity of intimate partner violence in the United States.

2. What was the purpose of this study? Why is this an important study to conduct?

3. What did the authors find? What characteristics made a woman more likely to be a victim of abuse? What were the common characteristics of abusive men in the study?

4. Comment on the role of the mental health of both the woman and her partner in intimate partner violence.

5. What are the implications of these findings for social workers and physicians working with women who have been victims of intimate partner abuse?

12

Smoking in the Movies Increases Adolescent Smoking: A Review

Annemarie Charlesworth and Stanton A. Glantz

ABSTRACT

Objective. Despite voluntary restrictions prohibiting direct and indirect cigarette marketing to youth and paid product placement, tobacco use remains prevalent in movies. This article presents a systematic review of the evidence on the nature and effect of smoking in the movies on adolescents (and others).

Methodology. We performed a comprehensive literature review.

Results. We identified 40 studies. Smoking in the movies decreased from 1950 to ~1990 and then increased rapidly. In 2002, smoking in movies was as common as it was in 1950. Movies rarely depict the negative health outcomes associated with smoking and contribute to increased perceptions of smoking prevalence and the benefits of smoking. Movie smoking is presented as adult behavior. Exposure to movie smoking makes viewers' attitudes and beliefs about smoking and smokers more favorable and has a dose-response relationship with adolescent smoking behavior. Parental restrictions on R-rated movies significantly reduce youth exposure to movie smoking and subsequent smoking uptake. Beginning in 2002, the total amount of smoking in movies was greater in youth-rated (G/PG/PG-13) films than adult-rated (R) films, significantly increasing adolescent exposure to movie smoking. Viewing antismoking advertisements before viewing movie smoking seems to blunt the stimulating effects of movie smoking on adolescent smoking.

Pediatrics, Dec 2005 v116 i6 p1516(13).
"Smoking in the Movies Increases Adolescent Smoking: A Review" by Annemarie Charlesworth and Stanton A. Glantz. ©2005 American Academy of Pediatrics

Conclusions. Strong empirical evidence indicates that smoking in movies increases adolescent smoking initiation. Amending the movie-rating system to rate movies containing smoking as "R" should reduce adolescent exposure to smoking and subsequent smoking.

INTRODUCTION

The tobacco industry has long recognized the value of smoking in movies to promote cigarettes and developed extensive programs to promote smoking in the movies. (1) After the US Congress held hearings on smoking in the movies in 1989 in response to the revelation that Philip Morris paid to place Marlboros in the film *Superman II*, the tobacco industry amended its voluntary advertising code (2) in 1990 to prohibit paid brand placement. In 1998, the tobacco industry signed the Master Settlement Agreement (MSA) with state attorneys general, which prohibited direct and indirect cigarette advertising to youth and paid product placement in movies. (3) Despite these agreements by the tobacco industry, the amount of smoking in the movies increased rapidly in the 1990s compared with the 1980s, reversing the downward trend that had existed since the 1950s and returning in 2002 to levels comparable with that observed in 1950 (4) (Fig 1). The Centers for Disease Control and Prevention attributed the slower-than-expected decline in adolescent cigarette use during

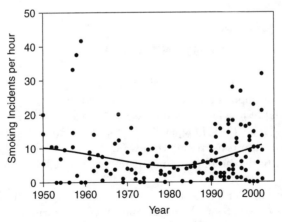

FIGURE 1 Smoking incidents per hour fell slowly through the 1950s through the 1980s and then increased rapidly beginning around 1990. By 2002, smoking intensity in movies had returned to the levels observed in 1950. (Redrawn from data in Glantz SA, Kacirk K, McColloch C. Back to the future: smoking in movies in 2002 compared with 1950 levels. *Am J Public Health.* 2004;94:261–263.)

the 1990s in part to the effects of smoking in the movies. (5,6) In recent years, there has been a wide range of research, including content analyses of films over time, focus groups, psychological experiments, and epidemiological studies on the effects of smoking in the movies, which, when taken together, provide strong and consistent empirical evidence that smoking in the movies promotes adolescent smoking.

METHODS

Using the search terms "smoking/tobacco" and "movies/films," we searched health, psychology, and social science databases (including PubMed, PsychInfo, and Eric) for research articles on smoking in the movies. We searched the Science Citation Index to find subsequent articles that cited the articles located in the initial searches, as well as following up citations in the articles that were located by using these 2 strategies. We also conducted a supplemental Internet search to locate unpublished research articles (nonindustry funded) regarding smoking in the movies, resulting in reports written by the American Lung Association, World Health Organization, Massachusetts Public Interest Research Group, and University of California, San Francisco Center for Tobacco Control, Research, and Education and a doctoral dissertation from the University of Melbourne. We did not limit our search to films produced within the United States, studies conducted within the United States, or studies conducted with certain age groups. This search resulted in a compilation of 40 studies.

CONTENT ANALYSES

We examined content analyses to determine the prevalence of tobacco (including actual or implied tobacco use, smoking advertisements, and paraphernalia) in samples of movies released between 1940 and 2002. Studies involved all top-grossing films (7–15) (generally the top 20 or 50 each year) or random samples drawn from top-grossing films. (4,16–22) Results did not seem to vary according to the sampling frame; therefore, they will be combined in the discussion.

Except for children's animated cartoons, which tended to feature more cigar use, (8,10) cigarettes are by far the most prevalent form of tobacco shown in movies. (11,13,17) A study of movies released each decade from 1940 to 1989 found that characters shown smoking in movies peaked in the 1950s. (19) The prevalence of smoking among major characters was substantially higher than among comparable (generally high socioeconomic status) people in the real world through the 1960s, 1970s, and 1980s. (16) The overall prevalence of smoking among major characters in movies was close to the levels observed in the general population (~25% in the 1990S). (19,23,24)

Magnitude of Smoking in Movies

A random sample of top-grossing films from 1950 through 2002 indicated that the amount of smoking (or other tobacco-related events) decreased from an average of 10.7 events per hour in 1950 to a low of 4.9 events per hour in 1980–1982 and then increased rapidly to 10.9 events per hour in 2002 (4,16,17,20,22) (Fig 1). (Other studies based on more intensive samples over shorter periods yielded similar results. (11,13,14)) Eighty-seven percent of popular films between 1988 and 1997 contained tobacco occurrences, with two thirds of those movies depicting tobacco use by ≥1 major character. (11) Almost half (46%) of the popular films from 1985 to 1995 featured at least 1 lead character who used tobacco. (18) Leading actors smoked in 60% of popular films from 2002 to 2003. (13) Although these different studies used different measures of smoking intensity, they consistently show that the pattern of smoking in movies does not mirror changes in the intensity of smoking in the actual population; between 1950 and 2000, adult smoking prevalence in the United States fell from 44% to 22.8%. (4)

Tobacco use in films in the 1980s and 1990s was not related to movie genre. (11,18) Tobacco use was rarely relevant to a scene and even less likely to be the major focus of the scene. In a sample of 1609 tobacco-use occurrences by major and minor characters in popular movies between 1988 and 1997, only 16.2% of occurrences were relevant to the scene, and only 5% were the major focus of the scene. (11)

Tobacco Presence According to Film Rating

The Motion Picture Association of America (MPAA) (the major film studios' lobbying organization) introduced its voluntary rating system on November 1, 1968, and has modified it several times since then (25) in response to public or congressional pressure. There are 5 ratings: G (general audiences, all ages admitted), PG (parental guidance suggested, some material may not be suitable for children), PG-13 (parents strongly cautioned, some material may be inappropriate for children under 13), R (restricted, under 17 requires accompanying parent or adult guardian), and NC-17 (no one 17 and under admitted).

Tobacco use remained stable in children's G-rated animated films from 1937 to 2000. (8,10) Disney films made after 1964 (when the first Surgeon General's report linked smoking to lung cancer (26)) contained similar rates of smoking to before 1964: at least 1 character in almost half of the films smoked. (8,10) Good and bad characters were equally likely to smoke. (8,10) Although the short-term negative health effects (ie, coughing) were depicted in some films (20% (8) or 37% (10) depending on the sample), none of the films depicted long-term health consequences. All children's animated feature films released from 1996 to 1997 depicted at least 1 character smoking. (8)

Until the mid-1990s, the number of smoking occurrences in films increased with the rating of the film, with R-rated movies featuring significantly more smoking than G-, PG-, or PG-13-rated films. (7,9,21,24) In films

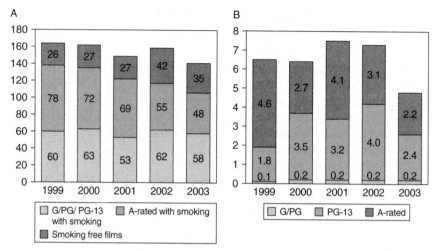

FIGURE 2   Beginning in 2002, more tobacco impressions were delivered to theatrical audiences in youth-rated (G/PG/PG-13) films than adult-rated (R) movies. A, Between 1999 and 2003, the number of youth-rated movies with smoking held steady, whereas the number of R-rated releases with smoking decreased 38%. B, The 20% drop in tickets sold from 2002 to 2003 (1.36–1.1 billion) accounts for 60% of the decline in tobacco impressions delivered by films in theatrical release. (This estimate does not include the number of impressions delivered through home video and broadcast television, which may have increased.) (Reproduced with permission from Polansky JR, Glantz SA. First-run smoking presentations in US movies 1999–2003. 2004. Available at: http://repositories.cdlib.org/ctcre/tcpmus/Movies2004.)

between 1988 and 1997, R-rated films featured significantly more tobacco use by major characters (81%) than G-rated (54.6%), PG-rated (53.1%), and PG-13-rated (64%) films. (11)

Beginning in the mid-1990s, the MPAA began to "down-rate" movies, (27) resulting in PG-13 ratings for many films that would have previously been rated R. This "ratings creep" also shifted the presentation of smoking incidents from mostly R-rated movies to teen-rated (PG-13) movies. (12,13,15) By 2002, youth-rated (G/PG/PG-13) movies delivered more tobacco impressions (1 person seeing tobacco use once) than R-rated movies (15) (Fig 2).

Character Tobacco Use and Motivation

The themes common to cigarette advertising (28) are common in movies. Smoking is routinely used to portray glamour, independence, rebelliousness, (20,22) relaxation or stress relief, (11,13,16,17,24) romance, (19) socializing or celebrating, (11,13,24) pensive thinking, and confiding in others. (11,24) In contrast to true smoking-prevalence patterns, which tend to be concentrated among people with lower socioeconomic status, (29) smoking movie characters are primarily male, white, and from upper socioeconomic brackets. (7,11,13,16–18,20) From the 1960s through the 1990s, the prevalence of smoking by major movie characters remained ~3 times that of comparable (high-socioeconomic-status) people in the actual population. (16,17)

Smoking is often portrayed with drinking (8,10,11) and other risky behaviors. (11)

There are gender differences in the portrayal of smoking. Male tobacco use is associated with violent behavior, dangerous acts, and gambling, whereas female tobacco use is associated with sexual affairs, illegal activities, and reckless driving. (11) Men were more likely to be depicted using tobacco to reinforce their masculinity, whereas women were more likely to be portrayed using tobacco to control emotions, manage stress, manifest power and sex appeal, enhance body image or self-image, control weight, or to give themselves comfort and companionship. (21) Various studies of movies made between 1960 and 1995 show strong majorities of male characters smoking. (16–18,20) Smoking among female leads nearly tripled from 11% in the 1960s to 30% in 1997. (16,17,20) An analysis of films released between 1993 and 1997 featuring the most popular female actresses (21) (aged 21–40 years) revealed that the rate of smoking lead or supporting characters were about the same for men (38%) and women (42%). Smoking was more common in movies starring younger actresses than older actresses; movies starring actresses in the youngest age quartile depicted 3.6 times more movie smoking incidents than movies featuring actresses in the oldest age group. (21)

Smoking in films is most commonly depicted as an adult behavior, with adolescents rarely depicted smoking (11,16); from 1988 to 1997, adolescents were depicted smoking in only 3.7% of smoking occurrences. (11)

Smoking is rarely presented realistically as an addiction that leads to disease and death or that causes anguish and suffering in smokers' families, (11,16,28) especially in films made for younger audiences. (21) Health messages related to tobacco use represented only 2% of tobacco events in the 1960s, 1% in the 1970s, and 4% in the 1980s. (16) In the top 25 US films released from 1988 to 1997, negative health, social, or legal consequences of smoking were depicted by only 3% (12 of 349) of the major characters using tobacco, and negative reactions to others using tobacco (such as negative comments or coughing) were depicted in only 6% of smoking occurrences. (11)

A World Health Organization report that examined the prevalence of smoking in Indian films and its impact on adolescents reported similar patterns of smoking in Indian movies as had been observed in US-produced movies. (30) Although cigarette smokers comprise only 14% of India's total tobacco-using population, tobacco use appeared in 76% of the films sampled, and cigarettes accounted for 72% of these incidents. As in the US, smoking was associated with stress reduction, rebellion, health, romance, popularity, and masculinity. Adolescents reported that they are influenced by smoking in the movies, because they wish to emulate the stars' behavior, and that off-screen smoking was equally as influential as on-screen smoking.

The fact that the presentation of smoking in the movies was rarely realistic and rather mirrored cigarette advertising themes was not coincidental. Internal tobacco-industry documents reveal extensive efforts by the tobacco industry not only to encourage product placement and smoking in movies but also to avoid negative portrayals. (1)

FOCUS GROUPS: HOW ADOLESCENTS PERCEIVE SMOKING IN THE MOVIES

Focus groups conducted in New Zealand (31,32) and Australia (33) examined how nonsmoking adolescents perceive and interpret smoking in movies. The results reflect what adolescents say about smoking in movies, not their responses to specific questions designed by adult researchers. Despite some differences in methods, their findings were consistent: both younger (12- to 13-year-old) and older (16- to 17-year-old) teens accepted smoking images as a reflection of everyday life, perceived smoking as a common and acceptable way of relieving stress, expressed a nonchalant attitude about the presence of smoking in movies and real life, and, although acknowledging health risks associated with smoking, still found smoking desirable. (31–33) These findings are consistent with tobacco patterns and use trends found in the content analyses.

Adult themes permeated adolescents' perceptions and attitudes about smoking, who saw smoking depictions as realistic. The prevalence of adult smoking in films (versus adolescent smoking) seems to reinforce stereotypes of adult behavior. Similarly, nonacceptance or judgment of smoking was regarded by adolescents as immature. (32) Adolescents did not consider movie smoking as influential on their behavior but expressed concern that "younger" children may be impressed, which may also reaffirm their desired "adult" self-image. (31,32) These findings suggest that adolescents do not smoke to look like other adolescents; they smoke to look like adults.

The unconscious acceptance of the smoking imagery in the movies is what may make it so powerful, (32) a fact long appreciated by the tobacco industry. (1) A 1972 letter from a movie production executive to RJ Reynolds Tobacco explained that "film is better than any commercial that has been run on Television or any magazine, because the audience is totally unaware of the sponsor involvement." (34)

EXPERIMENTAL STUDIES

Several experimental studies have examined the short-term effects of exposure to smoking in the movies on adolescents' and adults' attitudes and beliefs about smoking, smokers, (35–40) and intent to smoke. (35,38) The strength of experiments is that they provide data collected in a controlled environment, making it easier to draw causal conclusions. The weakness of the experiments is that it is only possible to assess effects on short-term outcomes such as attitudes in an artificial environment. These experiments, taken in the context of the other evidence, however, add substantially to the confidence we can have in the conclusion that smoking in the movies stimulates adolescent smoking. Consistent with the focus-group results, these studies found that exposure to movie smoking scenes made nonsmokers more tolerant and accepting of smoking and smokers and increased their likelihood of smoking in the future. (35–37,40)

Effects on Adolescents

To test the effects of movie smoking on nonsmoking adolescents' self-reported levels of positive arousal (emotional reactions) and beliefs about smokers, an experiment was conducted in which 9th-grade nonsmoking teens from California viewed movie scenes from 2 youth-oriented movies containing either the original scenes with smoking or professionally edited scenes with smoking removed without changing other content by simply reframing the image to remove the smoking. (35) (Students were allocated randomly to the different experimental groups.) Ninety-two percent of the adolescents accurately recalled seeing the smoking. These results confirmed a 1981 correspondence between the product-placement firm Associated Film Promotions and Brown and Williamson Tobacco that concluded that recall ability varied based on products and respondents under the age of 18 had the best overall recall rates and the highest recall for tobacco products. (1,41)

More important, smoking scenes, compared with nonsmoking scenes, elicited significantly more positive arousal, positively impacted beliefs about how a smoker's stature and vitality are perceived by others, and positively impacted beliefs about how smokers perceive their own stature. These findings suggest that smoking in movies evokes feelings of excitement and pleasure and weakens viewers' perceptions that smoking is socially objectionable. (35)

A study of Australian 7th- and 8th-grade students provided more details on how the portrayal of smoking by popular actors and actresses in selected 8-minute film clips affected student attitudes using a 2 × 2 × 2 design: (no smoking/smoking) × (low/high social status) × (protagonist/antagonist). (40) Although it did not reach statistical significance, there was a trend for students to perceive high rates of smoking prevalence in the population if they saw the video clips containing smoking regardless of the other experimental conditions. Viewing the high-status smoking characters was associated with more favorable attitudes toward smoking and higher smoking susceptibility; viewing the low-status characters smoking had the opposite effect. Regardless of the social status of the protagonist or antagonist, students who saw the protagonists smoke were more likely to think smoking would enhance their social stature, whereas students who saw antagonists smoke were more likely to think that smoking would detract from their social stature. These results are consistent with other studies suggesting that smoking in movies by characters with favorable social characteristics, which represent the vast majority of smoking presentations on screen, send a prosmoking message to adolescents.

Another experiment with nonsmoking 9th graders from California examined the effects of viewing an antismoking advertisement before a smoking movie. (35) For adolescents who did not see the antismoking advertisement, smoking scenes generated significantly more positive arousal, led to more favorable beliefs about a smoker's stature, and increased their intent to smoke. These effects were not found in adolescents who viewed an antismoking advertisement before movie smoking. Adolescents who saw the antismoking advertisement also had significantly more negative thoughts about the lead characters who were depicted as smokers. In addition, editing out the smoking did not affect adolescents' liking of the movie. Indeed, compared with a control advertisement (unrelated to smoking), showing the antismoking advertisement before both the smoking and nonsmoking versions of the movie significantly enhanced the adolescents' ratings of the film. (35)

These classroom-based findings were confirmed in an experiment conducted with the general public in a real theater. (42) In a survey conducted with female movie viewers (aged 12–17 years) as they left the theater, 48% of those who viewed an antismoking advertisement before a movie with smoking later responded that movie smoking was "not okay," compared with 28% of movie viewers who did not see the antismoking advertisement. Recall of the antismoking advertisement was greatest among the subjects who saw heavy smoking on screen. For current smokers, the antismoking advertisement had a significant effect on intention to smoke. Compared with smokers who did not see the antismoking advertisement, a significantly higher percentage of current smokers said they were unlikely to be smoking this time next year.

Effects on Young Adults and Adults

In studies conducted with young adults, identification with a smoking character seems to promote protobacco beliefs and attitudes and intent to smoke. As with adolescents, exposure to movie smoking is associated with adults' overestimation of smoking in real life. In a survey of Australian adults leaving theaters after the movie, more than half (52%) believed that smoking occurs more in real life than in the films; only 17% of the subject sampled believed that people in films smoke more than in real life. (39) Higher perceptions of smoking prevalence were associated with watching movies more frequently and lower educational status.

For smokers, exposure to movie smoking increased their desire to smoke, (38) likelihood to smoke in the future, (37,38) and perceived positive image of smoking. (36,37) Exposure to movie smoking also made nonsmokers more willing to become friends with a smoker (36) and increased their likelihood to smoke. (38) One study exposed smoking and nonsmoking undergraduate students to thematically similar 20 minute clips of the movie *Die Hard,* 1 with smoking and 1 without smoking. Compared with nonsmokers who viewed the nonsmoking clip, nonsmokers who viewed the smoking clip reported a greater willingness to become friends with a smoker. (36) Another study (38) asked smoking and nonsmoking undergraduate students to rate main movie characters from popular films on 12 dimensions, including sexiness, attractiveness, and popularity. One group rated characters in scenes with smoking and the other group rated the same characters in scenes in which they were not smoking. Viewing the smoking scenes increased the likelihood of future smoking by all participants and significantly increased male regular and occasional smokers' desires to smoke. (38)

Similar to the effects of viewing an antitobacco advertisement before viewing movie smoking on studies with California adolescents, (42,43) viewing antitobacco content in real movie theaters impacted Australian adults' attitudes about smoking and future intent to smoke. (39) Compared with subjects who saw a control movie (*Erin Brockovich*), those who saw a movie with antitobacco content (*The Insider*) showed a decline in intentions to smoke after the film regardless of whether they were current smokers, ex-smokers, or nonsmokers.

EPIDEMIOLOGICAL STUDIES

Epidemiological studies have been completed in 4 populations: California, (44,45) northern New England, (24,46–51) the entire United States, (52) and Victoria, Australia. (40) After controlling for other known risk factors for smoking initiation, cross-sectional (24,44,46–49) and longitudinal (45,50, 51,52) studies have demonstrated a strong dose-response relationship between the amount of movie smoking to which adolescents are exposed and the likelihood that they will begin smoking.

Effects of Total Exposure to Smoking in the Movies

The most direct assessment of the dose-response relationship between exposure to smoking in the movies and adolescent smoking was a cohort study of nonsmoking adolescents (aged 10–14 at study entry) in Vermont and New Hampshire, who were followed for 13 to 26 months. (50) After adjusting for covariates associated with adolescent smoking initiation, adolescents in the highest quartile of exposure to smoking in the movies were 2.71 times more likely to have started smoking than those in the lowest quartile of exposure. Fifty-two percent (95% confidence interval [CI]: 30% to 67%) of smoking initiation was attributable to exposure to smoking in the movies, a larger effect than that associated with cigarette advertising (34%). (53)

A national cross-sectional study (52) conducted in 2003 using the same methods as the New England longitudinal study (51) yielded statistically indistinguishable results. The national study included 6522 US adolescents aged

10 to 14 who agreed to participate in a random-digit-dialing telephone survey. After adjusting for covariates, adolescents in the highest quartile of exposure to smoking in the movies were 2.6 times more likely to have started smoking than those in the lowest quartile of exposure, with a dose-response relationship. In contrast to the New England study, (51) the national study did not show a significant interaction between parental smoking status and the effects of smoking in the movies; adolescents of smokers and nonsmokers were similarly sensitive to the amount of smoking in the movies.

The attributable risk fraction estimated from this national cross-sectional study (52) was 38% (95% CI: 20–56%). Although this point estimate is lower than the 52% estimate from the New England longitudinal study, the CIs for the 2 studies overlap and both include both point estimates. Aside from random variation, the point estimates may be different because of differences in the population baseline characteristics. In particular, all the subjects in the New England longitudinal study were nonsmokers at baseline, whereas some of the subjects were (by design) already smokers in the national cross-sectional study. Therefore, the 52% estimate from the longitudinal study may be a cleaner estimate of the point estimate of the attributable risk. In either case, the effect of smoking in the movies on adolescent smoking is substantial.

The effects of smoking in the movies are especially pronounced for children of nonsmoking parents (51) (Fig 3). High exposure to smoking in the movies can neutralize the effects of good (nonsmoking) parental role modeling. This observation is particularly relevant in terms of policy solutions to the problem of smoking in the movies. The MPAA, which controls the voluntary ratings system, states that its "primary task [is] giving advance cautionary warnings

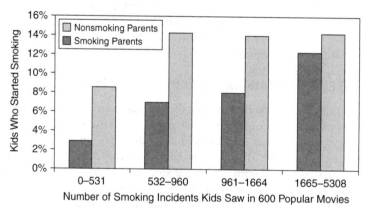

FIGURE 3   The effects of smoking in the movies are stronger in adolescents whose parents are nonsmokers than smokers. Indeed, heavy exposure to smoking in movies can negate the effects of good parental role modeling. The exposure ranges are quartiles of exposure to smoking in the movies. (Reproduced with permission from Stanton A. Glantz. Available at:
www.smokefreemovies.ucsf.edu/problem/now_showing.html.)

to parents so that parents could make the decision about the movie going of their young children." (54)

Effect of Favorite-Star Smoking

On-screen smoking by adolescents' favorite stars is another way to measure exposure to smoking in the movies. In films from 1994 to 1996, 65% of adolescents' favorite stars smoked in at least 1 film. (46)

A cross-sectional study (44) of 6252 California adolescents aged 12 to 17 examined the relationship between teens' smoking susceptibility and their favorite star's smoking status. After controlling for covariates related to adolescent smoking susceptibility, they found that stars favored by adolescent smokers and nonsmokers significantly differed, with adolescent smokers favoring stars who were more likely to smoke on screen. Nonsmoking adolescents who named a favorite star preferred by smokers were more likely to be susceptible to smoking (odds ratio [OR]: 1.35). (44)

In a follow-up longitudinal study (45) of 2084 California adolescents from the sample who were nonsmokers at baseline, adolescents whose favorite stars smoked on screen were significantly more likely to have smoked 3 years later. After controlling for confounding variables, adolescent girls whose favorite stars smoked in movies had increased odds of smoking compared with adolescents whose favorite stars did not smoke (OR: 1.86). When multivariate analysis was restricted to boys, receptivity to tobacco promotions, but not having a favorite star who smoked on screen, was related to smoking at follow-up. (45)

In a cross-sectional study of male and female adolescents in New England, the odds of having advanced smoking status and favorable attitudes toward smoking increased with the number of films in which their favorite star smoked. (46) Among never smokers, those who chose favorite stars who were smokers in films were much more likely to be susceptible to smoking (adjusted OR: 4.8 for stars who smoked in 2 films; OR: 16.2 for stars who smoked in $\geq$ 3 films). (46)

A cross-sectional study of 2610 students from Victoria, Australia, in grades 7 to 12 who had a favorite actor or actress did not detect any effect of on-screen smoking by the top 10 favorite actors or actresses on students' beliefs or intentions to smoke. (40) More important, however, this study found that on-screen smoking by favorite male actors was positively associated with student smoking behavior, especially among female students. On-screen smoking by favorite female actresses did not show an association with student smoking.

The California (44,45) and Australian (40) studies found that on-screen smoking had a stronger effect on girls than boys, whereas the New England (46,51) and US (52) studies found similar effects on both genders. The failure to find an effect of favorite stars on smoking by boys in California may reflect limitations in the way that the exposure measure was constructed. First, to be considered a smoker in the California study, a star had to smoke in at least

2 movies between 1994 and 1996. In contrast, the New England study classified the star as a smoker if he or she smoked in even 1 film. Hence, adolescents whose favorite stars smoked in only 1 movie in the New England study
would be counted as "unexposed" in the California study, which would potentially bias the results toward the null. Second, Pamela Anderson Lee, a Play-
boy playmate who appeared in the television series *Baywatch*, was listed as one
of the boys' favorite stars in the California study, whereas the New England
and Australian studies excluded her because her primary exposure was not in
films in theatrical release. The Australian study used a continuous measure of
the actual amount of smoking by the favorite actors and actresses and still
found different effects for boys and girls. It may be that the finding of greater
effect on girls may reflect the fact that girls prefer dramas, which contain more
smoking than action/adventure films (boys' general preference).

Preliminary studies (without controls for confounding) that examined
teens' media habits and smoking-related behaviors revealed that the more US
movies that Thai and Hong Kong teenagers had seen, the greater the likelihood of their having smoked. (55,56) For many of these teens, the desire to
emulate an American lifestyle led to smoking.

Measuring total exposure in terms of total number of smoking events is a
more complete and more sensitive measure of exposure than rates of favorite-
star smoking, because it captures all the exposure to smoking delivered to the
viewer. It is possible to have significant smoking in a film by someone other
than an adolescent's favorite star, but an adolescent seeing such a film would
be considered "unexposed" in the analysis of the relationship between movie
smoking exposure and adolescent smoking behavior. However, the fact that,
despite these limitations, the California study found an overall effect of fa-
vorite-star smoking is consistent with the conclusions from the New England
and national studies that the movies are having an effect on adolescent smoking behavior.

Relationship Between Reducing Exposure
and Adolescent Smoking Initiation

Given the dose-response relationship between exposure to smoking in the
movies and adolescent smoking initiation, one would predict that parental actions to reduce the "dose" would be associated with a reduction in adolescent
smoking. That prediction is correct. In the New England cohort, (51) exposure to movie smoking significantly decreased when parents increased restrictions on viewing R-rated movies. The reduced exposure to smoking was
accompanied by corresponding reductions in smoking initiation (14.3% of the
adolescents with little or no restrictions on viewing R-rated movies started
smoking, compared with 7.0% for those allowed to view R-rated movies once
in a while, and 2.9% for those never allowed to view them). As expected from
the result that the effects of smoking in movies had the largest effects in children of nonsmoking parents (Fig 3), parental restrictions on R-rated movies

had a greater impact in nonsmoking than smoking families. These findings also confirm those of earlier cross-sectional studies of the New England cohort that demonstrated that parental restriction of R-rated movies has a significant effect on exposure to movie smoking, (49) and that children with no restrictions or partial restrictions on R-rated movies were at greater risk for having tried smoking than those with complete restrictions. (48) Better enforcement of the R rating by parents and theaters could lead to a reduction in exposure to smoking in movies and, consequently, adolescent smoking.

The movie samples used in these epidemiological studies were collected from 1988 to 1997, when the majority of smoking presentations were in R-rated films. As a result, parental restriction on seeing R-rated films (presumably because of concern for language, violence, or sexual content) had a substantial effect in reducing adolescents' exposure to smoking in the movies. However, as of 2002–2003, most smoking depictions appeared in youth-rated (G/PG/PG13) rather than adult-rated (R) films. (12,13,15) This shift of smoking from R-rated films to youth-rated (mostly PG-13) films reduces the ability of parents who would choose to use the R rating as it was implemented in 2005 to reduce adolescent exposure to smoking in the movies. Modifying the rating system to rate smoking movies as R would permit both parents and theaters the opportunity to prevent adolescent smoking. (57)

TOBACCO USE IN MOVIES
AND TOBACCO-INDUSTRY RESTRICTIONS

The Voluntary Cigarette-Marketing Code

Coming under congressional scrutiny for both youth-targeted advertising and paid product placement in 1989, (1) the tobacco industry avoided legislative control of their marketing practices by modifying their voluntary cigarette-advertising and -promotion code in 1990 to indicate that "[n]o payment shall be made by any cigarette manufacturer or any agent thereof for the placement of any cigarette, cigarette package, or cigarette advertisement as a prop in any movie produced for viewing by the general public." (2) The pervasiveness of brand placements in youth- and adult-rated films, however, did not change after the tobacco industry's voluntary self-regulation. In 250 top-grossing US movies released from 1988 to 1997, (9) the frequency of tobacco brands remained stable. The type of tobacco brand appearance, however, changed after the tobacco industry's voluntary "ban" on brand placements: in films released before 1990, none contained both an actor using tobacco and background appearances (when the product's presence on screen was unrelated to characters' behavior). After 1990, 5% of films contained both actor use and background appearances, with actor use increasing from 1% to 11%. There were no differences in the frequency of brand appearances in films rated for adult versus adolescent audiences (35% vs 32%) before and after the ban (1988–1997).

The Master Settlement Agreement (MSA)

In 1998, 46 US state attorneys general settled the state lawsuits against the tobacco companies with the MSA. (3) In addition to paying money to the states
and accepting other restrictions on advertising, the cigarette companies agreed
that they would not "make or cause to be made, any payment or other consideration to any other person or entity to use, display, make reference to or
use as a prop any Tobacco Product, Tobacco Product package, advertisement
for a Tobacco Product or any other item bearing a brand name in any motion
picture, television show, theatrical production or other life performance, live
or recorded performance of music, commercial film or video, or video game."
(3) Although not a law, this agreement, unlike the 1990 cigarette-marketing
code, is a legally binding contract that could be enforced by a court. The
MSA, however, is probably not effective in preventing unbranded movie
smoking depictions (which probably would mostly benefit Philip Morris'
Marlboro, the leading children's cigarette) and would not prevent tobacco
companies from engaging in product-placement deals through their non-US
subsidiaries.

In its first 2 years, the MSA had little short-term effect on smoking or
tobacco-brand placements in youth-rated movies. A comparison of youth-
rated (PG-13) movies released in the 2 years before (1996–1997) and 2 years
after (1999–2000) the MSA showed that 80% of presettlement movies and
82% of postsettlement PG-13-rated movies contained tobacco use. In addition, the amount of screen time devoted to portraying tobacco increased by
50%, from an average of 0.89 minutes per film before the MSA to 1.35 minutes per film after it. (12) Brand placement in PG-13-rated movies continued
after the MSA. (12,58) The number of R-rated films with brand placements
released each year did fall after the MSA, but the number of PG-13-rated films
with brand display increased. (58) Although these findings may have resulted,
at least in part, from the mid-1990s trend to "down-rate" movies from R to
PG-13, (15,27) the fact remains that the level of exposure to tobacco in
adolescent-rated movies increased.

Although payment for tobacco placement in movies was supposed to have
ended in 1990, the tobacco industry found other approaches to promote smoking in movies beyond traditional product-placement deals that met the letter of
its voluntary advertising code. (1) This history suggests methods that a tobacco
company might use to work around the restrictions in the MSA. In addition to
formal product placement, strategies to increase tobacco's visibility and use in
entertainment media have included encouraging celebrity use and endorsement, sponsoring entertainment events, advertising in entertainment media,
and using the "glamour" associated with Hollywood in advertisement campaigns. (1) In addition, internal tobacco-industry documents reveal that movie
producers at times have eschewed check payments for product placement in
movies, preferring cash, jewelry, or other nontraceable forms of payment. (1)
Indeed, the tobacco industry has a long history of "working around" its agreements to limit its advertising and promotion activities. Analyses of cigarette

advertising since the inception of the tobacco industry's voluntary 1964 cigarette-advertising code and in succeeding years since its 1990 revision indicate that major provisions of the code have been routinely violated. (59,60)

The MSA also does not apply to payments for product placement by the non-US subsidiaries of the multinational tobacco companies, as was done when Philip Morris Europe (based in Switzerland) made an agreement with Pinewood Studios (in England) to place Marlboros in *Superman II* (1,61) or when Philip Morris' advertising agency (in Japan) worked through a Swiss intermediary to pay the London-based producers of the James Bond movie *License to Kill* $350 000 to feature Lark cigarettes as part of its effort to open up the Japanese market. (1,62,63) Both of these transactions could be executed today without violating the MSA. Smoking in the movies increased in youth-rated films despite the 1998 MSA prohibiting tobacco marketing to youth. A population-attributable risk calculation suggests that the movies account for ~390 000 new adolescent regular smokers in the United States annually, (53) enough to replace the 400 000 (64) active smokers that the tobacco industry kills every year. In addition, the distribution of movies featuring smoking to international audiences with even less public health protections than in the United States promises to recruit an untold number of young new smokers around the world.

CONCLUSIONS

Content analyses, focus groups, psychological experiments, and epidemiological studies provide a consistent chain of evidence that smoking in the movies leads adolescents to hold more protobacco attitudes and beliefs, which is consistent with the observed dose-response relationship between exposure to smoking in the movies and initiation of adolescent smoking. Movies teach children the same smoking stereotypes (glamour, coolness, attractiveness, sexiness, rebelliousness) and adult motivations (stress relief, celebration, romance) for smoking that pervade tobacco advertising and help establish the perception that smoking is normal, prevalent, and even desirable in society, especially among adults. The images of smoking in movies both normalize the behavior and downplay the negative health effects associated with smoking, encouraging more tolerant, neutral, or nonchalant attitudes about smoking. Although teens generally acknowledge the long-term health risks associated with smoking, they immediately experience the perceived short-term benefits of smoking, such as looking tough or sexy or fitting in with their peers, which reinforces and motivates adolescent smoking. (65) The overrepresentation of smoking in the movies with only positive outcomes contributes to adolescents' increased perceptions of smoking prevalence and the benefits of smoking and increases their likelihood of beginning to smoke. (66–68)

Movies are such a powerful influence on adolescents that they can negate the effects of positive parental role modeling on smoking (26) (Fig 3). Parental restrictions on viewing R-rated movies significantly reduced youth exposure to movie smoking and subsequent smoking. (51) As of 2005, >80% of PG-13- and R-rated movies contain smoking. As the movie industry shifts a greater share of their movies from the R to the PG-13 category, the smoking depictions contained in these movies become accessible to more adolescent viewers. This shift of smoking from R-rated movies to PG-13-rated movies reduces the effectiveness of parental R-rated movie restriction would have on adolescent smoking. Amending the ratings system to rate movies with smoking as R (as is done with strong language) would reverse the effects of ratings creep and substantially reduce adolescent exposure to smoking in movies. (An exception could be made for the few films that actually portray the negative consequences of smoking or a real historical figure who actually smoked, such as Winston Churchill). Because PG-13-rated films generally make more money than R-rated movies, producers would simply leave tobacco out of movies designed to be marketed to youth audiences, further reducing exposure. (57)

Such a policy change, as well as a requirement to disclose tobacco-industry involvement by the people involved in making a film (similar to the disclosures that are routinely required of people publishing articles in medical journals (69)), an end to brand identification, and antismoking advertisements run before movies containing tobacco use could substantially reduce the number of adolescents who begin smoking quickly, painlessly, and at low cost.

None of these policy changes would prohibit any content in a film or preclude artistic decisions by film makers. In particular, modernizing the MPAA's voluntary ratings system to treat smoking in the same way as "adult" language and rate new movies with smoking as R is not censorship. It would leave the free choice of whether to include smoking and accept an R rating with the producers and directors.

There are several opportunities for pediatricians to intervene to reduce the effects of smoking in the movies on their patients and children generally. They should educate them about the powerful effect that smoking in the movies has on children and encourage parents to enforce the R rating, because doing so reduces youth exposure to smoking in the movies and adolescent smoking initiation. As of March 2005, people can determine the tobacco-use status of films in theaters and on video at www.SmokeFreeMovies.ucsf.edu, www.SceneSmoking.org, and www.ScreenIt.com. Until the motion picture industry amends its voluntary ratings system to treat smoking in the same way that it treats offensive language and rates movies with smoking as R, parents can consult these Internet resources to determine which youth-rated movies include smoking and avoid those films.

In addition to encouraging individual action, pediatricians and the families who they serve can join organized efforts to advocate for the 4 policies described above. These policies, first advanced by the University of California Smoke Free Movies project (www.SmokeFreeMovies.ucsf.edu), have been endorsed by the American Academy of Pediatrics, among others. Because of the strong evidence of the linear dose-response relationship between smoking exposure and adolescent smoking, such policy changes would eventually reduce adolescent exposure (and initiation) by ~60%, preventing ~200 000 adolescents from starting to smoke each year and preventing ~62 000 premature deaths. (53)

From the Center for Tobacco Control Research and Education, Institute for Health Policy Studies, University of California, San Francisco, California. Accepted for publication Sep 1, 2005. doi:10.1542/peds.2005–0141

REFERENCES

1. Mekemson C, Glantz SA. How the tobacco industry built its relationship with Hollywood. *Tob Control.* 2002;11(suppl 1):i81–i91

2. Tobacco Institute. *Cigarette advertising and promotion code.* 1990. Available at: http://legacy.library.ucsf.edu/tid/nji49e00. Accessed October 12, 2005

3. National Association of Attorneys General. *Master Settlement Agreement; 1998.* Available at: www.library.ucsf.edu/tobacco/litigation/msa.pdf. Accessed October 12, 2005

4. Glantz SA, Kacirk K, McColloch C. Back to the future: smoking in movies in 2002 compared with 1950 levels. *Am J Public Health.* 2004;94:261–263

5. US Centers for Disease Control and Prevention. Trends in cigarette smoking among high school students: United States, 1991–2001. *MMWR Morb Mortal Wkly Rep.* 2002;51:409–412

6. US Centers for Disease Control and Prevention. Cigarette use among high school students: United States, 1991–2003. *MMWR Morb Mortal Wkly Rep.* 2004;53:499–502

7. Terre L, Drabman R, Speer P. Health-relevant behaviors in media. *J Appl Soc Psychol.* 1991;21:1303–1319

8. Goldstein AO, Sobol RA, Newman GR. Tobacco and alcohol use in G-rated children's animated films. *JAMA.* 1999;281:1131–1136

9. Sargent JD, Tickle JJ, Beach ML, Dalton MA, Ahrens MB, Heatherton TF. Brand appearances in contemporary cinema films and contribution to global marketing of cigarettes. *Lancet.* 2001;357:29–32

10. Thompson KM, Yokota F. Depiction of alcohol, tobacco, and other substances in G-rated animated feature films. *Pediatrics.* 2001;107:1369–1374

11. Dalton MA, Tickle JJ, Sargent JD, Beach ML, Ahrens MB, Heatherton TF. The incidence and context of tobacco use in popular movies from 1988 to 1997. *Prev Med.* 2002;34:516–523

12. Ng C, Dakake B. *Tobacco at the Movies: Tobacco Use in PG-13 Films.* Boston, MA: Massachusetts Public Interest Research Group Education Fund; 2002

13. American Lung Association-Emigrant Trails. *The thumbs up! thumbs down! annual ten year report on tobacco in the movies: 1994–2003.* Sacramento, CA: American Lung Association; 2003

14. Mekemson C, Glik D, Titus K, et al. Tobacco use in popular movies during the past decade. *Tob Control.* 2004;13:400–402

15. Polansky JR, Glantz SA. *First-run smoking presentations in US movies 1999–2003.* 2004. Available at: http://repositories.cdlib.org/ctcre/tcpmus/Movies2004. Accessed March 20, 2005

16. Hazan AR, Lipton HL, Glantz SA. Popular films do not reflect current tobacco use. *Am J Public Health.* 1994;84:998–999

17. Stockwell TF, Glantz SA. Tobacco use is increasing in popular films. *Tob Control.* 1997;6:282–284

18. Everett SA, Schnuth RL, Tribble JL. Tobacco and alcohol use in top-grossing American films. *J Community Health.* 1998;23:317–324

19. McIntosh W, Bazzini D, Smith S, Wayne S. Who smokes in Hollywood? Characteristics of smokers in popular films from 1940 to 1989. *Addict Behav.* 1998;23:395–398

20. Stockwell TF, Glantz SA. Smoking in movies remained high in 1998. *Tob Control.* 1998;7:441–442

21. Escamilla G, Cradock AL, Kawachi I. Women and smoking in Hollywood movies: a content analysis. *Am J Public Health.* 2000;90:412–414

22. Kacirk K, Glantz SA. Smoking in movies in 2000 exceeded rates in the 1960s. *Tob Control.* 2001;10:397–398

23. Omidvari K, Lessnau K, Kim J, Mercante D, Weinacker A, Mason C. Smoking in contemporary American cinema. *Chest.* 2005;128:746–754

24. Valenti J. *Movie ratings: how it all began.* Available at: www.mpaa.org/movieratings/about. Accessed March 20, 2005

25. United States Department of Health Education and Welfare. *Smoking and health: report of the Advisory Committee to the Surgeon General of the Public Health Service.* 1965. Available at: http://profiles.nlm.nih.gov/NN/B/B/M/Q/_/nnbbmq.pdf. Accessed October 12, 2005

26. Sargent JD, Dalton MA, Beach ML, et al. Viewing tobacco use in movies: does it shape attitudes that mediate adolescent smoking? *Am J Prev Med.* 2002;22:137–145

27. Thompson KM, Yokota F. Violence, sex, and profanity in films: correlation of movie ratings with content. *MedGenMed.* 2004;6:3

28. US Federal Trade Commission. *U.S. Federal Trade Commission Staff Report on the Cigarette Advertising Investigation.* Washington, DC: US Federal Trade Commission; 1981

29. Centers for Disease Control and Prevention. Cigarette smoking among adults: United States, 2002. *MMWR Morb Mortal Wkly Rep.* 2004;53:427–431

30. World Health Organization. *Hollywood: Victim or Ally? A Study on the Portrayal of Tobacco in Indian Cinema.* Geneva, Switzerland: World Health Organization; 2003

31. McCool JP, Cameron LD, Petrie KJ. Adolescent perceptions of smoking imagery in film. *Soc Sci Med.* 2001;52:1577–1587

32. McCool JP, Cameron LD, Petrie KJ. Interpretations of smoking in film by older teenagers. *Soc Sci Med.* 2003;56:1023–1032

33. Watson NA, Clarkson JP, Donovan RJ, Giles-Corti B. Filthy or fashionable? Young people's perceptions of smoking in the media. *Health Educ Res.* 2003;18:554–567

34. Richards R. *We are about to go into production with the motion picture, "Run Sheep Run," a suspense, thriller, set in Los Angeles.* 1972. Available at: http://legacy.library.ucsf.edu/tid/ylm89d00. Accessed October 12, 2005

35. Pechmann C, Shih C. Smoking scenes in movies and antismoking advertisements before movies: effects on youth. *J Mark.* 1999;63:1–13

36. Gibson B, Maurer J. Cigarette smoking in the movies: the influence of product placement on attitudes toward smoking and smokers. *J Appl Soc Psychol.* 2000;30:1457–1473

37. Dal Cin M, Fong G, Gibson B, Zanna M. *Smoking characters in movies increases automatic identification with smoking: an experimental study using implicit measures [abstract].* Presented at: Society for Research on Nicotine and Tobacco Annual Meeting; February 18, 2003: New Orleans, LA.

38. Hines D, Saris RN, Throckmorton-Belzer L. Cigarette smoking in popular films: does it increase viewers' likelihood to smoke? *J Appl Soc Psychol.* 2000;30:2246–2269

39. Dixon HG, Hill DJ, Borland R, Paxton SJ. Public reaction to the portrayal of the tobacco industry in the film The Insider. *Tob Control.* 2001;10:285–291

40. Dixon H. *Portrayal of Tobacco Use in Popular Films: An Investigation of Audience Impact* [PhD thesis]. Melbourne, Australia: University of Melbourne; 2003

41. Associated Film Promotions. *Recall and recognition of commercial products in motion pictures.* 1981. Available at: http://legacy.library.ucsf.edu/tid/hgo30f00. Accessed October 12, 2005

42. Edwards C, Harris W, Cook D, Bedford K, Zuo Y. Out of the Smokescreen: does an anti-smoking advertisement affect young women's perception of smoking in movies and their intention to smoke? *Tob Control.* 2004;13:277–282

43. Pechmann C. A comparison of health communication models: risk learning versus stereotype priming. *Media Psychol.* 2001;3:189–210

44. Distefan JM, Gilpin EA, Sargent JD, Pierce JP. Do movie stars encourage adolescents to start smoking? Evidence from California. *Prev Med.* 1999;28:1–11

45. Distefan JM, Pierce JP, Gilpin EA. Smoking in movies influences adolescents to start smoking: a longitudinal study. *Am J Public Health.* 2004;94:1–6

46. Tickle JJ, Sargent JD, Dalton MA, Beach ML, Heatherton TF. Favourite movie stars, their tobacco use in contemporary movies, and its association with adolescent smoking. *Tob Control.* 2000;10:16–22

47. Sargent JD, Beach ML, Dalton MA, et al. Effect of seeing tobacco use in films on trying smoking among adolescents: cross sectional study. *BMJ.* 2001;323:1394–1397

48. Dalton MA, Ahrens MB, Sargent JD, et al. Relation between parental restrictions on movies and adolescent use of tobacco and alcohol. *Eff Clin Pract.* 2002;5:1–10

49. Sargent JD, Dalton MA, Heatherton TF, Beach ML. Modifying exposure to smoking depicted in movies. *Arch Pediatr Adolesc Med.* 2003;157:643–648

50. Dalton MA, Sargent JD, Beach ML, et al. Effect of viewing smoking in movies on adolescent smoking initiation: a cohort study. *Lancet.* 2003;362:281–285

51. Sargent JD, Beach ML, Dalton MA, et al. Effect of parental R-rated movie restriction on adolescent smoking initiation: a prospective study. *Pediatrics.* 2004;114:149–156

52. Sargent JD, Beach ML, Adachi-Mejia AM, et al. Exposure to movie smoking: its relation to smoking initiation among US adolescents. *Pediatrics.* 2005;116:1183–1191

53. Glantz SA. Smoking in the movies: a major problem and a real solution [published correction appears in Lancet. 2004;363:250]. *Lancet.* 2003;362:258–259

54. Motion Picture Association of America. *The birth of the ratings.* 2004. Available at: www.mpaa.org/movieratings/about/index.htm. Accessed October 12, 2005

55. Goldberg M. American media and the smoking-related behaviors of Asian adolescents. *J Advert Res.* 2003;43:2–11

56. Goldberg M, Baumgartner H. Cross-country attraction as a motivation for product consumption. *J Bus Res.* 2002;55:901–906

57. Glantz SA. Rate movies with smoking "R." *Eff Clin Pract.* 2002;5:31–34

58. Adachi-Mejia AM, Dalton MA, Gibson, JJ, et al. Tobacco brand appearances in movies before and after the Master Settlement Agreement. *JAMA.* 2005;293:2341–2342

59. Richards JW Jr, Tye J, Fischer PM. The tobacco industry's code of advertising in the United States: myth and reality. *Tob Control.* 1996;5:295–311

60. Pollay RW. Promises, promises: self-regulation of US cigarette broadcast advertising in the 1960s. *Tob Control.* 1994;3:134–144

61. Spengler P. *"Superman II": the movie.* 1979. Available at: http:// legacy.library.ucsf.edu/tid/cxz55e00. Accessed October 12, 2005

62. Lambert A, Sargent JD, Glantz SA, Ling P. How Philip Morris unlocked the Japanese cigarette market: lessons for global tobacco control. *Tob Control.* 2004;13:379–387

63. Danjaq SA. *[Regarding License to Kill].* 1988. Available at: http:// legacy.library.ucsf.edu/tid/bbs24e00. Accessed October 12, 2005

64. Centers for Disease Control and Prevention. Annual smoking-attributable mortality, years of potential life lost, and economic costs: United States, 1995–1999. *MMWR Morb Mortal Wkly Rep.* 2002;51:300–303

65. Halpern-Felsher B, Biehl M, Kropp R, Rubinstein M. Perceived risks and benefits of smoking: differences among adolescents with different smoking experiences and intentions. *Prev Med.* 2004;39:559–567

66. Alesci N, Forster J, Blaine T. Smoking visibility, perceived acceptability, and frequency in various locations among youth and adults. *Prev Med.* 2003;36:272–281

67. Perkins H, Meilman P, Leichliter J, Cashin R, Presley C. Misperceptions of the norms for the frequency of alcohol and other drug use on college campuses. *J Am Coll Health.* 1999;47:253–258

68. US Department of Health and Human Services. *Preventing tobacco use among young people: a report of the Surgeon General.* 1994. Available at: www.cdc.gov/tobacco/sgr/ sgr_1994/#Major%20Concl. Accessed October 12, 2005

69. Krimsky S, Rothenberg L. Financial interests and its disclosure in scientific publications. *JAMA.* 1998;280:225–226

DISCUSSION QUESTIONS

1. What was the purpose of this study?

2. What method did the researchers employ in this study?

3. What were the results of the content analysis? How was smoking portrayed in the movies?

4. What were the results of the experimental studies?

5. What sort of policy changes do the authors recommend to combat the effect of smoking in the movies? Do you think this would be effective?

13

Binge Drinking During the First Semester of College: Continuation and Desistance From High School Patterns

Alan Reifman and Wendy K. Watson

ABSTRACT

Students' first semester on campus may set the stage for their alcohol use/misuse throughout college. The authors surveyed 274 randomly sampled first-semester freshmen at a large south-western university on their past 2 weeks' binge drinking, their high school binge drinking, and psychosocial factors possibly associated with drinking. They conducted separate analyses among high school nonbinge drinkers (testing for predictors of college binge onset vs continued nonbinge drinking) and high school binge drinkers (testing for predictors of continued binge drinking in college vs desistance from drinking). In both analyses, the variables that predicted college binge drinking largely revolved around gregarious socializing (eg, partying, having a social network of individuals who drank relatively heavily). Gender was predictive only among high school nonbinge drinkers; women had a higher probability than did men of adopting binge drinking in college.

Journal of American College Health, Sept–Oct 2003 v52 i2 p73(9)
"Binge Drinking During the First Semester of College: Continuation and Desistance From High School Patterns" by Alan Reifman and Wendy K. Watson. © 2003 Heldref Publications

INTRODUCTION

Heavy drinking by college students has been found to be associated with student deaths and injuries, sexual abuse, and school dropout. (1) In an address at the National Press Club on August 26, 1999, Penn State University President Graham Spanier cited binge drinking among 5 issues that pose challenges to American higher education. (2) Nationally representative studies from the Harvard School of Public Health by Wechsler and colleagues (1) that were conducted between 1993 and 2001 have consistently shown the prevalence of binge drinking (consumption at a single sitting within the last 2 weeks of 5 or more drinks in a row for men, 4 or more for women) to be high—approximately 45%.

For all the interest in college students' drinking, researchers have rarely focused on the heavy consumption that students often start before they arrive on campus. In one of Wechsler and colleagues' studies of college students' drinking, (3) respondents were asked retrospectively about their binge drinking during high school. Findings revealed great continuity between high school and college drinking patterns. Sixty nine percent of the sample exhibited consistency between their high school and college binge drinking (47% not binge drinking in either high school or college and 22% binge drinking at both levels). The remaining respondents (32%) could be considered to have exhibited a change: 22% did not binge in high school but started to drink heavily in college, whereas 10% were binge drinkers in high school but not in college (numbers do not add to 100%, presumably because of rounding). Leibsohn's (4) study of freshman students at a Midwestern university showed an even greater continuity: 86% of respondents kept the same pattern of getting or not getting drunk from high school to college. Leibsohn concluded that: "By the time students enter college their drug and alcohol patterns are well established" (p190).

These demonstrations of considerable high school to college continuity of drinking patterns clearly suggest that a key element in reducing the prevalence of binge drinking in college students is prevention at much earlier ages. But that does not mean that health educators at the college level are helpless in their efforts to prevent alcohol misuse. Although students who exhibit changes from high school to college (either taking up or giving up binge drinking) represent well below half of all students when applied to all collegians in the United States, the actual numbers of students who could be affected might easily reach into the hundreds of thousands or even millions.

Following this line of argument, health educators would be in a position to intervene with both high school nonbinge drinkers (to prevent them from taking up binge drinking in college) and with high school binge drinkers (to get them to give up binge drinking). We can cite several reasons for focusing on the first semester of college. First, Wechsler and colleagues' (5) national binge-drinking prevalence studies have indicated that college freshmen, sophomores, juniors, and seniors have similar rates of binge-drinking prevalence. One potential explanation for this similarity is that once students establish a pattern of drinking during the first year of college, they may tend to maintain it for the remaining years on campus. A second reason is that university personnel who can provide health education information probably have their greatest access to students during this period. Virtually all schools probably have some form of orientation for new students that includes extensive contact between staff and students, and some schools require first-year students to live in residence halls. That encourages contact between resident assistants and students. After students move off campus for their later years of college, school personnel probably have less access to them.

To develop intervention strategies that prevent high school nonbinge drinkers from beginning binge drinking in college and to get high school binge drinkers to abandon this behavior, health educators should know the psychosocial factors that are associated empirically with transitions in student drinking behavior. In this study, we seek to identify such factors separately in subgroups of high school nonbinge drinkers and binge drinkers. Among the variables we examined in this study are those traditionally used in alcohol research, including demographic factors (eg, gender, race), attitudes, alcohol expectancies, and potential social influences (eg, peer drinking, fraternity/sorority membership).

In an examination of concurrent (ie, cross-sectional) relationships between binge-drinking status (yes/no) and numerous predictor variables, Wechsler and colleagues (6) found several significant results. White students had greater odds of binge drinking than did non-Whites, and men had higher odds than did women. Among the strongest predictors were items that asked students how important they felt it was to engage in different activities while in college. Students who stated that "parties" were important, and "religion" not important, were most likely to be binge drinkers. Living in a fraternity or sorority house greatly increased the odds of binge drinking.

Leibsohn's study, (4) which focused on the transition to college, included 1 analysis that examined only college students who had used a substance in the previous month. Those students were asked with whom they had used alcohol or other drugs since coming to the university. Of students who had gotten drunk, 36% reported doing so exclusively with new friends, and another 57% reported doing so with new and old friends. Noted Leibsohn, "The overall trend was that very quickly most entering freshmen found new friends with whom they could get drunk and do drugs." (4) (p186) Peer influences thus remain an important area for study.

Weitzman et al (7) used the 1999 Harvard national study to examine the uptake of binge drinking among college freshmen. They confined analyses for this particular study to respondents who had not been high school binge drinkers. In their final multiple-predictor model, these authors found several individual and social factors (eg, White race, membership in a Greek organization, perception of heavy drinking among friends) to predict the onset of binge drinking with significant accuracy. We used similar predictors in the present study. Weitzman et al also examined environmental factors (eg, the price students pay for alcoholic beverages) that we did not examine in this study, although environmental influences are an important area for prevention that we address later.

Baer and colleagues (8) also studied the transition from high school to college, but their sample consisted solely of "high-risk" students (identified partly on the basis of their engaging in a heavy-drinking episode while in high school). Being male and living in fraternity/sorority residences were associated with increased drinking from high school to college. The studies by Weitzman and colleagues (7) and Baer and colleagues (8) appear to complement each other—one study focused on first-year college students who had refrained from heavy drinking while in high school, whereas the other focused on those who had been heavy drinkers. Because the Baer et al study used only a small number of predictors, the 2 studies are not highly comparable. Yet, both reported that Greek involvement was an important predictor. We included both high school nonbinge drinkers and binge drinkers in this study.

Our objective was to identify psychosocial factors that predict college binge drinking separately in subgroups of high school nonbinge drinkers and binge drinkers as a means of facilitating preventive efforts at the college level with both of these groups. At a general level, we hypothesized that college students (whether high school nonbinge drinkers or heavy drinkers) who possess or come into contact with the risk factors reviewed above (eg, male gender, Greek involvement, high valuation of partying, belonging to heavy drinking social networks) would be most likely to engage in binge drinking during their first semester at the university.

METHOD

Sample

We surveyed a random sample of freshmen who lived in residence halls who entered Texas Tech University during the 1999 fall term, their first semester of college. Given the nature of random sampling and the university's requirement that first-year students live in the residence halls (with some allowable exceptions), the sample in theory can be considered largely representative of first-year students at the university as a whole. Freshmen who lived in the residence hall system on or around the first day of classes in fall 1999 totaled 3,283. To achieve our goal of sending out 600 questionnaire packets, we used systematic sampling with a random start. (9) Written materials in the packet alerted students that the project would involve 3 waves of measurement for which they were offered payments of $10, $10, and $20 for completing the respective waves (wave 2 took place in spring 2000, and wave 3 during fall 2000).

We received approval for the study from the Institutional Review Board (IRB) at Texas Tech University. Our present study used data only from wave 1 to maintain the focus on the transition to college and also because of college officials' presumed greater access to students at that time. Data from waves 2 and 3 will be used for longitudinal analyses of drinking trends and predictor variables' temporal precedence in relation to student drinking.

We distributed wave-1 questionnaire packets in mid-October 1999, after students had been in school for approximately a month and a half. The staff of the central housing office initially delivered all packets in the individual residence halls. Because of some slight differences in the timing of each hall's receipt of its packets, plus differences among students in how rapidly they returned their questionnaires, we received completed questionnaires between October 20 and December 1. Differences in arrival time were unrelated to students' drinking levels. (10)

We retained participants' names because of the payment aspect of the study and the need to link each respondent's survey answers over time for longitudinal analyses. To protect confidentiality, we implemented standard procedures (eg, retention of all information in a locked office, use of identification numbers, no listing of names in research data files). The consent form contained assurances to students that these steps would be taken, that data would be used only for research, and data would be reported in the aggregate only.

We collected data from 274 respondents at wave 1–174 women (63.5%) and 100 men (36.5%). Because women were overrepresented in our sample and men were underrepresented, compared with Texas Tech's roughly 50/50 gender composition, and because the genders differed somewhat in their binge-drinking levels, we analyzed the data with sample weights designed to equalize the proportion of men and women. Under that approach, 45.6% of the overall sample were binge drinkers according to the Wechsler definition of binge drinking (5 drinks in a row at a single sitting for men and 4 for women) compared with the figure of 44.7% that is obtained when no special weighting by gender is used (ie, the original proportions of men and women are left alone). Because of this great similarity and for simplicity, we conducted all the remaining analyses in this article without sample weights. In terms of race/ethnicity, 235 (86%) wave-1 respondents were White, 22 (8%) were Hispanic, 8 (3%) were Black, 7 (2.6%) were Asian/Pacific Islanders, 1 was a Native American/Alaskan Native, and 1 was considered other/unknown (each of the latter 2 made up less than 1% of the sample).

That the wave-1 response rate was below 50% concerned us. However, when we made follow-up reminder calls and obtained other information, we learned that at least 23 students could not reasonably be expected to return the questionnaire: 10 students apparently dropped out of school during the study period (indicated by disconnected telephone numbers and/or questionnaire packets returned unopened); 3 students were under 18 and thus ineligible to participate; 1 was a second-year student (the study was restricted to first-year students); and 9 students claimed they did not receive a packet until too close to the ending deadline for us to send them replacement packets (16 other students whose lack of a questionnaire we learned about in time were sent replacement packets). Thus, we estimate that our wave-1 participation rate was 274/577 = 47%. (One completed survey was returned by a student who claimed to be beyond the first year of college, although she lived in a residence hall with and was a friend of freshmen students. Results were virtually identical whether or not the student was included in the data analyses. The results reported here include the student.) Other college studies have also obtained approximately 50% participation rates, (11) so that the present return rate, especially with a mail survey, is not out of line.

Ultimately, however, a randomly drawn sample, such as we had, is not necessarily the same as a representative sample when there is a substantial rate of nonparticipation. Our gender proportions are an illustration of the nonrepresentativeness of our sample. It is possible that heavy drinkers and individuals with other characteristics were underrepresented at wave 1, although our lack of data on wave-1 nonparticipants precludes a direct comparison. Attrition analyses using data from students who were in the study at wave 1 revealed that those who did not remain in the study at wave 2 tended to be heavier drinkers than those who did remain. (10) If nonparticipation in an initial wave and attrition of initial participants at a later wave represent the same underlying dynamic, heavy drinkers probably were underrepresented at wave 1, but we do not know whether that was the case. Note, however, that before their attrition at wave 2, a number of heavy drinkers were known to have been in the sample at wave 1, arguing perhaps that wave-1 participants represented a sizable range of drinking levels.

Measures

Participants completed a 2-part survey instrument. The first part, 117 items, consisted of a set of standard closed-ended measures to which the students responded on a Scantron computer-scorable form. The second part included a grid for listing information about one's social network. Because the network grid is somewhat complex, we felt it was not suited to using the Scantron, therefore the students wrote their answers directly on it.

Binge Drinking

Whether the student had engaged in at least 1 heavy-drinking or binge episode in the last 2 weeks was our dependent variable. Two items assessed the number of binge-drinking episodes in the last 2 weeks as defined by Wechsler and colleagues. (3) One item pertained to 5+ drink episodes for men and the other to 4 drinks for women. We combined the 2 items into a single variable of number of binge-drinking episodes in the last 2 weeks so that each respondent had the proper gender-specific value. For this study, we dichotomized respondents' number of binge episodes into zero versus one or more. We took these items directly from Wechsler and colleagues (3) to ensure comparability of our binge-drinking rates to those reported by other investigators in other samples. (A recent special issue of the journal *Psychology of Addictive Behaviors* (12) was devoted to examining the strengths and limitations of using the 5/4-drink criterion of binge drinking; we encourage interested readers to consult it.)

Two similar, additional items asked respondents to report on their heavy-drinking episodes (5+ and 4 drinks) in a "typical" 2-week period during the students' senior year of high school. Thus, the high school binge-drinking measure was retrospective, rather than in "real time." We used this variable to separate the sample into high school binge drinkers and nonbinge drinkers.

Variables used to predict respondents' drinking transitions from high school to college can be grouped into several sets. Readers should recall that we assessed these variables during the first semester of college, concurrent with the college binge-drinking measure. For the most part, therefore, they do not offer prospective prediction of college binge drinking, except perhaps for demographic variables that are stable characteristics of the individual respondent.

Demographics

Respondents indicated gender, race/ethnicity (later collapsed into White/non-White), area lived in during high school (urban, suburban, rural), how they have been spending their weekends during the semester (always staying on or around campus, sometimes staying on campus and sometimes going home, always going home), and the educational attainment of each parent (< high school diploma through doctorate or professional degree). Previous studies of adolescent and young adult substance use suggest that these types of variables might have predictive value in this study. (13–15)

The questionnaire asked whether the respondent was a member of a fraternity or sorority (yes/no) and whether he or she intended to join one but had not yet done so. We believed that the latter question would be helpful in detecting self-selection effects (ie, whether people with certain drinking patterns are prone to join Greek organizations; students at the university where we conducted this study cannot live in fraternity or sorority houses). Living in a fraternity or sorority house is a bigger risk factor for binge drinking than being a member but not living in the house, according to the Harvard School of Public Health study. (5,16)

Lifestyle Importance

Following the lead in one of the studies by Wechsler and colleagues, we asked students how important it was for them to participate in 6 activities (parties, religion, athletics, community service, arts, and academics) that were scored from not at all important (0) to very important (3).

Perceived Friends' Approval
of Drinking Behaviors (Norms)

Respondents were asked how they thought their friends would respond (from strong disapproval [0] to strong approval [6]) if they knew that the respondent had engaged in 4 alcohol-related behaviors (drank alcohol every weekend, drank alcohol daily, drove a car after drinking, drank enough alcohol to pass out). (17) Item scoring was from 1 to 7 in the original source, but in this and other instances, we made zero the low point to coincide with the Scantron answer forms and averaged the items into an index with the internal consistency reliability coefficient $\alpha = .84$.

Alcohol Expectancies

We used 4 subscales (each of 5 items) from the Alcohol Effects Questionnaire (AEQ) (18) to measure respondents' beliefs about the effects they expected alcohol to have on them. The domains assessed, a sample item from each one, and the alpha reliability are as follows: social and physical pleasure (SPP; "Drinking makes me feel good"; $\alpha = .73$); sexual enhancement (SEX; "I often feel sexier after I've had a few drinks"; $\alpha = .77$); relaxation and tension reduction (REL; "Alcohol decreases muscular tension in my body"; $\alpha = .56$); and cognitive and physical impairment (IMP; "I'm more clumsy after a few drinks"; $\alpha = .75$). Respondents indicated whether they thought each item was true (1) or false (0). We averaged the items in a subscale; the resulting number represented the percentage of items the respondent had endorsed. Respondents who had never consumed alcohol were asked to answer these items with reference to how they thought it would affect them. These respondents were included in the analyses the same as everyone else, with no special treatment or statistical adjustment. Even if their expectancies were not based on direct drinking experience for some respondents, but rather came from outside sources (eg, seeing other people who had been drinking or a television/movie depiction of drinking), they could still potentially affect behavior.

Emotional Well-Being

We used the Positive and Negative Affect Schedule (PANAS) to obtain separate measures of positive and negative feelings. (19) Each scale consisted of 10 single-word emotion items. Respondents indicated the extent to which they had felt each emotion in the last 2 weeks (from very slightly or not at all [0] to extremely [4]). Examples of the positive affect items were excited, strong, and proud ($\alpha = .89$); negative items were distressed, upset, and jittery ($\alpha = .86$).

Party School Perceptions

We asked respondents, "During the time you were deciding where to go to college, to what degree did people give you the impression Texas Tech is a 'party school'?" Options ranged from not at all (0) to a great deal (9).

Romantic Relationship

Respondents used yes and no to indicate whether they currently had a romantic relationship.

Social Network Members' Drinking

We gave respondents a network grid on which to list (by initials) up to 8 people they considered members of their social network, using a question to elicit respondents' networks that was based on that used by Hays and Oxley (20) in their college-student study. The key terms in this question required that the respondents consider people with whom they have contact—at school, at work, at home, or in social or religious setting; that respondents consider relationships with potential network members to be enjoyable or worthwhile; and that respondents have seen the person since the start of the college semester. The network instrument also asked respondents to provide information on 13 attributes of each network member (eg, gender, length of time they have known the member, how close the respondents felt to the member). For each attribute, one or more summary indices could be derived (eg, percentage of men or women in the network).

Of the 13 attributes measured on the network grid, we used only that related to respondents' perceptions of network members' drinking. We asked respondents to characterize the drinking of each network member according to the following scale: abstainer (1); occasional/light social drinker (2); moderate/average social drinker (3); frequent/heavy social drinker (4); problem drinker (5); alcoholic (6); don't know (7). This network drinking question parallels a measure used by Leonard and colleagues. (21) We calculated an average of the network's drinking (excluding "don't-know" responses) for each respondent, the only network-based variable we used in the present study.

Age at First Drunkenness

We asked respondents, "How old were you the first time you got drunk or very high from alcohol?" (with an option to indicate that one had never been drunk). To create a meaningful ordinal variable that took into account people who had never been drunk, we created a trichotomous variable. We classified respondents under one of 3 descriptions: early (age $\leq$ 14 years) onset of drunkenness (1), late (ages 15–19 years) onset of drunkenness (2), and never been drunk (3). Higher scores thus meant progressively delayed onset and presumably less risk of future problems. We based the item and scoring scheme on work by Thomas and colleagues (22) and used this variable only in the analysis of high school binge drinkers to predict their continuation of or desistance from binge drinking in college.

Because high school nonbinge drinkers may never in their lives have been drunk or may have experienced their first drunkenness in college, we felt that the age of drunkenness onset variable might be somewhat confounded with the dependent variable of whether the students binged in college, so we did not use it in this group. We acknowledge that measures of self-reported drunkenness are not necessarily interchangeable with other measures of heavy drinking, such as the 5/4-drink measure, given that different individuals can become intoxicated after consuming different numbers of drinks. Age at first drunkenness is not necessarily interchangeable with grade level at first drunkenness (although some might consider the latter equally important); however, age and year of school are likely to be highly correlated.

RESULTS

Preliminary Descriptive Statistics

We conducted a 2 × 2 cross-tabular analysis to examine respondents' status in high school (no, yes) and college binge drinking (no, yes). The data in Table 1 indicate that approximately 75 % of the students' binge-drinking patterns remained consistent from high school to college (41% of the sample did not binge in either high school or college, and 34% binged in both). This relatively high degree of statistical association between high school and college binge-drinking status is apparent in the Cramer's V statistic of .48 (values can range from 0 to I) and a significant chi-square test, χ^2 (1, N = 272) = 63.85, p < .001. This high rate of continuity from high school to college matches those found by Wechsler and colleagues (3) and Leibsohn. (4) Evidence in the table also indicates that, overall, approximately 45% of the students in our sample engaged in binge drinking during their first semester of college (combining the students who did and did not binge in high school), which is similar

TABLE 1   Students' Binge-Drinking Status During High School and During the First Semester of College (Past 2 Weeks)

	Binge Drinking			
	College			
	No		Yes[†]	
High school	n	%	n	%
No	111	41	30	11
Yes[†]	40	15	91	34

Note. Percentages are for the full sample; they do not sum to 100% because of rounding.
χ^2(1, N = 272) = 63.85, p < .001, Cramer's V = .48.
[†] "Yes" refers to 1 or more binge episodes (men, 5 drinks, women 4 drinks at one sitting).

to national binge-drinking rates for freshmen and for college students as a whole found by Wechsler and colleagues. (5)

Main Analysis Plan

Essentially, we conducted 2 completely separate investigations: one examined high school nonbinge drinkers only, with whether these students binged in college as the dependent variable. This analysis could help determine factors associated with high school nonbinge drinkers' becoming binge drinkers in college or continuing to refrain from such conduct. The second set of analyses dealt with high school binge drinkers only, again with college binge drinking as the dependent variable, which could help determine factors associated with high school binge drinkers' continuing their binge drinking in college or desisting from such behavior.

Initially, we performed logistic regression analyses separately in the high school nonbinge and binge samples to examine which of the predictor variables were related to the dichotomous college (first semester) binge-drinking variable. Approximately 25 predictor variables were in each equation, with all of them entered as one block (ie, we did not use stepwise procedures that iteratively add and remove predictors). We then examined predictors that were significant in the logistic regression analyses individually, using two-way (College Binge Drinking × Predictor) chi-square analyses, to simplify presentation of the results. Only these chi-square results are shown in this article; a report on the logistic regression analyses is available from the authors. The value of the initial logistic regression analyses is that they allowed the relation of each predictor variable to the dependent variable to be examined while controlling for all other predictors in the models; the logistic regression analyses thus served as a useful gatekeeper for the later chi-square analyses.

High School Nonbinge Sample

On the basis of the results of the logistic regression analysis for the high school nonbinge sample, we retained the following significant predictor variables for the chi-square analyses: Alcohol Expectancies of Social and Physical Pleasure (SPP), average drinking of the social network, party importance, perceived friends' approval of drinking (norms), and gender.

In the logistic regression analyses (unless inherently categorical, eg, gender), we used continuous versions of the predictor variables. For the chi-square tables, however, these significant continuous predictors had to be converted into categorical form. The AEQ-SPP subscale included items that asked respondents whether they endorsed 5 purported pleasurable aspects of alcohol (it makes one feel good, has a pleasant taste, adds warmth to social occasions, is a good way to celebrate, and promotes joining people in enjoyable situations). The categories in the chi-square analyses for SPP thus represented the proportion of the 5 items that the respondents endorsed (ie, one category is .00, the other is .20). For average network drinking, we created a categorical variable using cut points such as 1.00–1.99, 2.00–2.99, because these numerical values can be linked to the original rating scale of network member drinking (ie, 1 = abstainer, 2 = occasional or light social drinker). For party importance, we intended to use the original response choices (not at all important to very important) as categories in the chi-square analysis, but few respondents endorsed the option of very important, so we merged it with one of the other choices to create the category of important or very important. Finally, because the Likert-type response scale for perceived friends' approval/norms for drinking did not have the same kind of concrete reference points as did the network drinking items, we divided the friend approval index scores into low, medium, and high by splitting the distribution as close as was possible into thirds (ie, cutting near the thirty-third and sixty-seventh percentiles).

Chi-square analyses are shown in Table 2. Each section displays a two-way frequency table (college binge drinking [none vs ≥ 1 time] by a categorical predictor variable), the associated chi-square test, and the value of Cramer's V. With the exception of gender, all chi-square analyses were significant at $p < .001$ and the Cramer's V values were all fairly large (from .37 to .44). The top section shows the relationship between expectations of alcohol's producing social and physical pleasure (AEQ-SPP) and college binge drinking. The greater the number of pleasurable alcohol-related aspects respondents endorsed, the more likely those high school nonbinge drinkers were to have taken up binge drinking in college. By looking specifically at the extreme groups on AEQ-SPP, we can see the dramatic nature of this relationship: Among high school nonbinge drinkers who endorsed none of alcohol's purportedly pleasurable effects, there was a zero probability of their taking up binge drinking in college (as of the time of the college drinking assessment we used). However, among those high school nonbinge drinkers who endorsed all of the pleasurable features of alcohol, 45% began binge drinking in college.

In Table 2, the section headed average network drinking shows the relationship between the average drinking of a student's network members and his or her binge drinking in college; respondents whose networks had scores from 1.00–1.99 (indicating that the networks contain at least some, if not mostly or entirely, abstainers) were extremely unlikely to begin binge drinking in college. As the average drinking of the networks increased, so did the likelihood of the respondents' initiating binge drinking in college. (Because extremely heavy drinking networks were rare among the high school nonbinge drinkers, we defined the final category of network drinking as 3.00 and above.)

The more these high school nonbinge drinkers felt that parties were an important aspect of college participation (Table 2, party importance) and the more they perceived their friends to approve of drinking behaviors (Table 2, friend approval), the greater their likelihood of adopting binge drinking during their first semester of college. An interesting trend in each case was that

TABLE 2 Two-way Frequencies of College First-Semester Binge Drinking and Predictor Variables Among High School Nonbingers Only

	College Binge Drinking (past 2 wk)		
Variable	No Binge	≥1	Probability of ≥1 Binge
AEQ-SPP score			
.00	26	0	.00
.20	18	1	.05
.40	21	4	.16
.60	17	6	.26
.80	17	10	.37
1.00	11	9	.45

AEQ-SPP = Alcohol Effects Questionnaire–Social and Physical Pleasure; the higher the scores, the greater the belief that alcohol increases pleasure.
$\chi^2(5, N = 140) = 21.28$, $p < .001$; Cramer's $V = .39$.

Average network drinking			
1.00–1.99	72	4	.05
2.00–2.99	31	18	.37
≥3	7	8	.53

Respondents rated drinking of each network member on a scale from abstainer (1) to alcoholic (6); scores were averaged for each respondent.
$\chi^2(2, N = 140) = 27.68$, $p < .001$; Cramer's $V = .44$.

Party importance			
Not at all	65	4	.06
Somewhat	35	19	.35
Important/very important	11	7	.39

$\chi^2(2, N = 141) = 19.44$, $p < .001$; Cramer's $V = .37$.

Friend approval of drinking			
Low	68	4	.06
Medium	33	19	.37
High	10	7	.41

$\chi^2(2, N = 141) = 21.87$, $p < .001$; Cramer's $V = .39$.

Gender			
Male	41	6	.13
Female	70	24	.26

$\chi^2(1, N = 141) = 3.05$, $p = .08$; Cramer's $V = .15$.

the main difference in probability of college binge drinking appeared between the lowest and middle categories of the predictor variable; the probability of binge drinking did not increase greatly between the middle and highest categories of the predictor.

Gender was another significant predictor in the overall logistic regression analysis but was only marginally significant in the chi-square follow-up. Among high school nonbinge drinkers, women had a higher probability of taking up binge drinking in college than did men (Table 2, gender). The Cramer's V associated with the chi-square analysis was .15.

High School Binge Sample

On the basis of the logistic regression analysis for the high school binge sample, we retained 2 predictors for follow-up chi-square analyses: average network drinking and party importance. The two-way frequencies (College Binge Drinking × Predictor), chi-square tests, and Cramer's V values for network drinking, and party importance are shown in Table 3. Paralleling the analyses with the high school nonbinge sample, we also found that greater average network drinking (V = .52) and greater importance attached to parties (V = .36) in the high school binge sample were both associated with higher probabilities of respondents' engaging in college binge drinking.

TABLE 3 Two-way Frequencies of College First-Semester Binge Drinking and Predictor Variables Among High School Binge Drinkers Only

	College Binge Drinking (past 2 wk)		
Variable	No Binge	≥1	Probability of ≥1 Binge
Average network drinking			
1.00–1.99	13	0	.00
2.00–2.99	21	54	.72
≥3	6	37	.86

Respondents rated drinking of each network member on a scale from abstainer (1) to alcoholic (6); scores were averaged for each respondent.
$\chi^2(2, N = 131) = 35.38, p < .001$; Cramer's V = .52.

Party importance			
Not at all	7	4	.36
Somewhat	27	41	.60
Important/very important	6	45	.88

$\chi^2(2, N = 130) = 16.78, p < .001$; Cramer's V = .36.

COMMENT

The findings in this study reveal some similarities and differences in the variables that predict college binge drinking among high school nonbinge drinkers and binge drinkers. Among high school nonbinge drinkers, significant predictors of the adoption of college binge drinking included expectancies of social and physical pleasure from alcohol, heavy drinking by one's social network, feeling that it was important to participate in parties, the perception that one's friends approved (or at least did not strongly disapprove) of various drinking behaviors, and being a woman. Among high school binge drinkers, significant predictors of the persistence of college binge drinking again included the variables network drinking and party importance.

With the exception of gender, the significant predictors appear to form a constellation around the theme of gregarious socializing with friends. All 4 variables (social and physical pleasure expectancies, network drinking, party importance, and friends' approval of drinking) correlated with each other from .41 to .54 in the full sample. These correlations suggest some degree of conceptual overlap, although this did not prevent variables from independently predicting college binge drinking among the high school nonbinge drinkers and/or binge drinkers. One might also expect the Greek-involvement variables to overlap with belonging to heavy-drinking social networks. However, the 2 Greek-involvement variables (membership and intention to join) each correlated with average network drinking only .14; although these correlations were statistically significant ($p < .05$), their magnitudes are probably lower than one might have expected. That the Greek-involvement variables did not predict binge drinking in either of the groups also could have resulted from the assessment of Greek involvement's having taken place too early in the first year to be relevant.

These findings can be placed in a better context when one looks at the transition to college more generally. This transition appears to contain elements of both positive and negative affect. According to Pancer and colleagues, (23) "The majority of students who are about to enter university appear to approach this transition in their lives with feelings of joy and anticipation. . . . In the weeks and months leading up to their first classes at university, they envision a life free of parental control, filled with interesting and novel activities, new people to meet, and stimulating academic work" (p 38). Hays and Oxley (20) further reported that within the first few weeks of college, among dormitory residents at least, students are busy forming social networks that consist heavily of new acquaintances. This is consistent with the idea that new students are devoting great time and energy to socializing with their fellow students.

As Pancer and colleagues (23) also pointed out, things may quickly become more stressful because of students' being away from home, having to do their own household tasks, and facing more demanding academic material than that to which they had been accustomed, conditions that could lead to alcohol use in an attempt to cope. What is striking about the present findings is that college binge drinking appears to be related principally to variables tapping into the exuberant/gregarious side of college life and not related to the distressing side (negative affect was not a significant predictor of college binge drinking in either the high school nonbinge drinkers or binge drinkers).

For the high school nonbinge drinkers only, the remaining predictor of college binge drinking was female gender. Much, if not most, research on adolescent drinking has found that male students drink more heavily than female students do. Our finding should be taken with caution because of its small statistical magnitude and the likeliness of self-selection of respondents in corresponding to the different participation rates of women and men. Replication of this gender difference in initiation of binge drinking is necessary if readers and researchers are to have greater confidence in it.

Limitations

Although our study had some strengths, including a randomly drawn sample, it also had some limitations, primarily that we assessed the predictors during the first semester of college, largely concurrently with the college binge drinking measure (although high-school binge drinking was reported retrospectively). Thus, this research design does not offer a prospective prediction of college binge drinking, except perhaps for demographic variables that are stable characteristics of the respondent. We cannot, therefore, determine the direction of causality of many relationships between variables.

We also gathered data during the second semester of the students' first year of college and the first semester of the sophomore year, which may ultimately allow us to gain a better sense of causal directionality. The study reported here, however, was designed to focus on the unique period of the initial transition to college.

Our reliance on self-reported drinking is also a potential limitation, although this practice is widespread in alcohol research and appears to have satisfactory validity. (3) Respondents' estimates of their network members' drinking could suffer from additional limitations; respondents probably would not witness all the drinking their network members do and the respondents' own drinking levels could color their estimates of others' drinking. (24) A final limitation is that the initial logistic regression models may have been vulnerable to overfitting (ie, retention of extra, unnecessary predictors resulting from the large number of predictor variables we used).

The present findings, as well as others in the literature, appear to have implications for preventing heavy drinking in college students. College health educators must find ways to take advantage of their access to new students on campus. New-student orientations may provide one important opportunity. Although many universities appear to deliver some form of alcohol-prevention message during orientation sessions, the University of Puget Sound (UPS) appears to have one of the more systematic and multifaceted programs of using the beginning of the school year for alcohol prevention. (25) Specifically, UPS provides a workshop during new-student orientation from counseling, health, and wellness services (CHWS); alcohol education outreach from the student development office during residence halls' first meetings of the year; and CHWS presentations to parents during orientation and parent/family weekend.

Prevention ideas must target students' peer relations and apparent sense of gregariousness in binge drinking. New students' natural desires to socialize with their fellow students cannot (and should not) be suppressed. The key will be to channel these activities in directions that do not involve heavy drinking. Although a great deal of discussion in college-drinking prevention circles mentions the need for schools to offer nonalcohol alternative activities for students' participation and entertainment, evaluative research data are scarce; some commentators have expressed skepticism about the ultimate effectiveness of nonalcohol activities. One promising program that does have some data is Late Night Penn State, a series of movies, musical performers, and comedians. Penn State has conducted surveys about the program and reports that as of February 2000, 46% of students said they attended at least one Late Night event. (26) A large majority of students who attended one late night event claimed that this reduced their own drinking and said they believed that the program reduced drinking among attendees. In an assessment of reasons for not attending Late Night, only 4% of those who gave reasons for not attending the event said it was "because alcohol is not available."

An additional prevention focus, suggested by Weitzman and colleagues, (7) is availability of alcohol in the college environment. These investigators found that variables such as students' perceived easy access to alcohol and cheap prices for it predicted onset of binge drinking in college. Weitzman et al suggested that "the potential significance to prevention of access, price—and place-related variables may be great. Unlike variables describing family history and/or peers, they are under the control of schools and communities" (p34).

In conclusion, further creativity on the part of college administrators and health educators, accompanied by empirical evaluative data, may lead the way toward reduced levels of heavy drinking in college students' socializing activities.

REFERENCES

1. Wechsler H, Wuethrich B. *Dying to Drink: Confronting Binge Drinking on College Campuses*. Emmaus, PA: Rodale; 2002.

2. Spanier GB. *Remarks to National Press Club*. August 26, 1999. Available at: http://www.psu.edu/ur/presspass/SpanierNPC.html.

3. Wechsler H, Davenport A, Dowdall G, Moeykens B, Castillo S. Health and behavioral consequences of binge drinking in college: a national survey of students at 140 campuses. *JAMA*. 1994;272:1672–1677.

4. Leibsohn J. The relationship between drug and alcohol use and peer group associations of college freshmen as they transition from high school. *J Drug Education*. 1994;24:177–192.

5. Wechsler H, Lee JE, Kuo M, Seibring M, Nelson TF, Lee H. Trends in college binge drinking during a period of increased prevention efforts: findings from 4 Harvard School of Public Health College Alcohol Study surveys: 1993–2001. *J Am Coil Health.* 2002;50:203–217.

6. Wechsler H, Dowdall GW, Davenport A, Castillo S. Correlates of college student binge drinking. *Am J Public Health.* 1995;85:921–926.

7. Weitzman ER, Nelson TF, Wechsler H. Taking up binge drinking in college: the influences of person, social group, and environment. *J Adolesc Health.* 2003;32:26–35.

8. Baer JS, Kivlahan DR, Marlatt GA. High-risk drinking across the transition from high school to college. *Alcohol Clin Exp Res.* 1995;19:54–61.

9. Babbie E. *The Practice of Social Research.* 8th ed. Belmont, CA: Wadsworth; 1998.

10. Reifman A, Watson W, McCourt A. *Social Networks and Heavy Drinking in College Students* (Technical Report). Texas Tech University. Available at: http://www.hs.ttu.edu/research/reifman. Accessed June 20, 2000.

11. Reifman A, Dunkel-Schetter C. Stress, structural social support, and well-being in university students. *J Am Coil Health.* 1990;38:271–277.

12. Carey KB, ed. Special issue: Understanding binge drinking. *Psychol Addict Behav.* 2001; 15(4).

13. Reifman A, Barnes GM, Dintcheff BA, Farrell MP, Uhteg L. Parental and peer influences on the onset of heavier drinking among adolescents. *J Stud Alcohol.* 1998;59:311–317.

14. Results related to alcohol use in different types of localities (ie, urban, rural). *Substance Abuse and Mental Health Services Administration. National Household Survey on Drug Abuse.* Available at http://alcoholism.about.com/library/ndkpat21.htm and http://www.samhsa.gov/oas/facts/alcoholuse.htm. Accessed March 6, 2002.

15. Wills TA, McNamara G, Vaccaro D. Parental education related to adolescent stress-coping and substance use: development of a mediational model. *Health Psychol.* 1995;14:464–478.

16. Honan WH. Study ties binge drinking to fraternity house life. *New York Times.* December 6, 1995:16.

17. Baer JS. Effects of college residence on perceived norms for alcohol consumption: an examination of the first year in college. *Psychol Addict Behav.* 1994;8:43–50.

18. Rohsenow DJ. Drinking habits and expectancies about alcohol's effects for self vs others. *J Consult Clin Psychol.* 1983;51:752–756.

19. Watson D, Clark LA, Tellegen A. Development and validation of brief measures of positive and negative affect: the PANAS scales. *J Pers Soc Psychol.* 1988;54:1063–1070.

20. Hays RB, Oxley D. Social network development and functioning during a life transition. *J Pers Soc Psychol.* 1986;50:305–313.

21. Leonard KE, Kearns J, Mudar P. Peer networks among heavy, regular and infrequent drinkers prior to marriage. *J Stud Alcohol* 2000;61:669–673.

22. Thomas G, Reifman A, Barnes GM, Farrell MP. Delayed onset of drunkenness as a protective factor for adolescent alcohol misuse and sexual risk taking: a longitudinal study. *Deviant Behav.* 2000;21:181–210.

23. Pancer SM, Hunsberger B, Pratt MW, Alisat S. Cognitive complexity of expectations and adjustment to university in the first year. *J Adolesc Res.* 2000;15:3–57.

24. Marks G, Graham JW, Hansen WB. Social projection and social conformity in adolescent alcohol use: a longitudinal analysis. *Pers Soc Psychol Bull.* 1992;18:96–101.

25. University of Puget Sound. *Alcohol prevention and education activities*. June 24, 2002. Available at: http://www.ups.edu/dsa/Alcohol_EDU.htm. Accessed May 16, 2003.

26. Pennsylvania State University, Student Affairs. *Late Night Penn State*. February 2000. Available at: http://www.sa.psu.edu/sara/pulse/late_night_69.shtml. Accessed March 14, 2002.

DISCUSSION QUESTIONS

1. Why were the authors interested in studying the drinking behavior of college students in the first trimester of college?

2. What were the authors' predictions for this study?

3. What were the results for high school non-binge drinkers (i.e., what were the significant predictors of college binge drinking for these students)?

4. What do the authors speculate is the main reason that college students engage in binge drinking?

5. What are the implications of these findings for encouraging college students to drink in moderation?

14

The Role of Self-Objectification in the Experience of Women with Eating Disorders

Rachel M. Calogero, William N. Davis, and J. Kevin Thompson

ABSTRACT

Objectification theory has linked self-objectification to negative emotional experiences and disordered eating behavior in cultures that sexually objectify the female body. This link has not been empirically tested in a clinical sample of women with eating disorders. In the present effort, 209 women in residential treatment for eating disorders completed self-report measures of self-objectification, body shame, media influence, and drive for thinness on admission to treatment. Results demonstrated that the internalization of appearance ideals from the media predicted self-objectification, whereas using the media as an informational source about appearance and feeling pressured to conform to media ideals did not. Self-objectification partially mediated the relationship between internalized appearance ideals and drive for thinness; internalized appearance ideals continued to be an independent predictor of variance. In accordance with objectification theory, body shame partially mediated the relationship between self-objectification and drive for thinness in women with eating disorders; self-objectification continued to be an independent predictor of variance. These results illustrate the importance of understanding and

Sex Roles: A Journal of Research, Jan 2005 v52 i1–2 p43(8).
"The Role of Self-Objectification in the Experience of Women With Eating Disorders" by Rachel M. Calogero, William N. Davis, and J. Kevin Thompson. © 2005 Plenum Publishing Corporation

targeting the experience of self-objectification in women with eating disorders or women at risk for eating disorders.

INTRODUCTION

Sexual objectification occurs whenever a person is viewed, evaluated, reduced to, and/or treated by others as merely a body, and has been identified as especially harmful to women (Bartky, 1990; Fredrickson & Roberts, 1997; Kaschak, 1992). Objectification theory considers self-objectification to be an adaptive strategy for girls and women who live in a culture that sexually objectifies the female body (Fredrickson & Roberts, 1997). The term self-objectification refers to the psychological process by which women internalize observers' objectifying perspectives on their bodies and become chronic self-monitors of their own physical appearance. This form of self-perception allows women to anticipate, and thus to exert some control over, how others treat them.

By coming to view their own bodies through this objectified lens, women engage in a kind of psychologically distancing from their physical bodies, which in turn contributes to negative attitudes toward and experiences with their bodies. This experience of self-objectification has been theoretically and empirically linked to a variety of negative consequences in nonclinical samples of adult and adolescent women, including increased opportunities for experiencing body shame, anxiety, negative attitudes toward menstruation, a disrupted flow of consciousness, diminished awareness of internal bodily states, depression, sexual dysfunction, and disordered eating (Calogero, 2004; Fredrickson, Roberts, Noll, Quinn, & Twenge, 1998; Noll & Fredrickson, 1998; Roberts, 2004; Slater & Tiggemann, 2002; Tiggemann & Slater, 2001).

Self-objectification may be a critical factor to identify for the treatment and recovery of women with eating disorders. This form of self-perception has not been examined empirically in a clinically eating disordered population, where disconnection and distancing from the body is prominent. Eating disorders have been described, in part, as women's response to feeling powerless to control the systematic objectification of their bodies (Fredrickson & Roberts, 1997). An exploration of the role of self-objectification in this population of women may provide information about the cultural construction of eating disorders that extends beyond fat phobia to include broader sociocultural forces.

To begin, it is necessary to consider what specific factors might contribute to the experience of self-objectification in women with eating disorders. Fredrickson and Roberts (1997) theorized that the virtually unavoidable exposure to sexualized depictions of female bodies and body parts in the visual media is a major contributor to this form of self-perception. Recently, researchers have demonstrated that reading contemporary woman's magazines for appearance-based and gender role advice was positively related to objectifying one's own body and accepting the content of the messages (Kim & Ward,

2004). A meta-analytic review of 43 tests of the immediate impact of exposure to the thin beauty ideal produced a small but consistent and significant effect size (Groesz, Levine, & Murnen, 2002), which demonstrates that the visual media also contribute to experiences of negative body image. Based on a review of various research designs and methodologies, Stice (2001) has suggested that the negative effects of media exposure could be considered a causal risk factor for eating disturbances.

Several dimensions of the media's potential influence on women's beliefs about and behavior toward their bodies have been examined recently in nonclinical and clinical eating disordered samples (Calogero, Davis, & Thompson, 2004; Thompson, van den Berg, Roehrig, Guarda, & Heinberg, 2004). These dimensions include the degree to which media are considered important sources of information about appearance, feeling pressured by media to conform to ideal standards, and internalizing general and athletic body ideals. A clinical sample of 440 eating disordered inpatients scored higher across almost all dimensions of media influence than did a nonclinical sample of 380 college students. The one exception was the dimension that measured the importance of the media as an informational source about appearance, where the nonclinical sample was slightly higher or roughly equivalent to the clinical sample.

Thus, the first purpose of the present study was to examine which dimensions of media influence, if any, predict self-objectification among women in a residential eating disordered population. The second purpose was to examine whether there was a direct or indirect relationship between dimensions of media influence and eating disorder pathology, with self-objectification as the hypothesized mediator, among women in a residential eating disordered population. A cardinal feature of eating disorders is some degree of caloric restriction and excessive concern with weight (American Psychiatric Association, 1994; Bruch, 1973, 1982). To approximate the assessment of this feature of eating disorders pathology, a measure of drive for thinness was utilized.

Next, the contribution of self-objectification itself to experiences of body shame and disordered eating in women with eating disorders was considered. Recurrent opportunities for women to experience body shame in both public and private contexts are powerful motivators to engage in disordered eating. Noll and Fredrickson (1998) demonstrated that body shame mediated the relationship between self-objectification and disordered eating behaviors in nonclinical samples, and they found that both predictors contributed independently to the variance in disordered eating. Similarly, women with eating disorders may behave in unhealthy ways in an attempt to alleviate feelings of shame about the body or, by self-objectifying, to avoid the experience of shame altogether. Thus, the final purpose of the present study was to examine whether there is a direct or indirect relationship between self-objectification and eating disorder pathology, with body shame as the hypothesized mediator, among women in residential treatment for eating disorders. Again, drive for thinness was utilized as the measure of eating disorders pathology in this model.

METHOD

Participants

Participants were 209 women in a residential treatment facility for women with eating disorders. Only patients who provided research consent upon admission were included in the present study. Patients were diagnosed on the basis of a semi-structured interview by a senior staff psychiatrist using criteria from the *Diagnostic and Statistical Manual of Mental Disorders* (4th ed., American Psychiatric Association, 1994). In this sample, 31.2% were diagnosed with anorexia nervosa restricting subtype (ANR; n = 69), 13.7% with anorexia nervosa-binge-purge subtype (ANBP; n = 27), 35% with bulimia nervosa (BN; n = 70), and 20.2% with eating disorder not otherwise specified (EDNOS; n = 43). Mean body mass index (BMI) was 19.70, and mean age was 22.90 years. Ninety-five percent of the women were European American, 1.8% were African American, 1.8% Asian, and 1.4% marked unspecified "other."

Measures

Self-Objectification Questionnaire. The Self-Objectification Questionnaire (SOQ; Fredrickson et al., 1998; Noll & Fredrickson, 1998) assesses the extent to which individuals view their bodies in observable, appearance-based terms versus nonobservable, competence-based terms without an evaluation of how satisfied they are with their bodies. Participants rank ordered 10 body attributes by how important each was to their own physical self-concept from 0 (least impact) to 9 (greatest impact). Difference scores were computed by subtracting the sum of the 5 competence attributes (e.g., health, strength) from the sum of the 5 appearance attributes (e.g., physical attractiveness, weight). Scores ranged from -25 to 25; higher scores indicate greater self-objectification. Consistent with objectification theory, self-objectification scores were uncorrelated with BMI in this sample ($r = .05$, ns). Satisfactory construct validity has been shown elsewhere (Noll & Fredrickson, 1998).

Body Shame Questionnaire. The Body Shame Questionnaire (Fredrickson et al., 1998) assesses the phenomenological aspects of body shame that occur when individuals imagine looking at themselves in the mirror. This indirect measure of shame circumvents the difficulty of eliciting accurate responses from individuals who may feel ashamed of being ashamed. Participants rated 18 items comprising motivational and behavioral components of shame (e.g., "I wish I were invisible," "I feel like crawling into a corner") using a 5-point Likert scale from 1 (not at all) to 5 (extremely). Scores ranged from 18 to 90; higher scores indicate greater body shame when looking at oneself in the mirror. Cronbach's alpha indicated high internal consistency across the 18 items ($\alpha = .95$).

Sociocultural Attitudes Toward Appearance Scale-3. The Sociocultural Attitudes Toward Appearance Scale-3 (SATAQ-3; Thompson et al., 2004) is a 30-item questionnaire that assesses four dimensions of media influence on body image and eating disturbances: information, pressures, internalization—general, and internalization—athletic. The information dimension includes 9 items that measure the degree to which various media are important sources for obtaining information about attractiveness and fashion (e.g., "Magazine articles are an important source of information about fashion and being attractive"). The pressures dimension includes 7 items that measure the degree to which individuals have felt pressured by various media to change their appearance (e.g., "I've felt pressure from TV and magazines to lose weight"). The general internalization dimension includes 9 items that measure the degree to which individuals have "bought into" the norms for body shape and weight portrayed in the media and the degree to which they attempt to match these standards by modifying certain behaviors (e.g., "I would like my body to look like the people who are on TV"). The athletic internalization dimension includes 5 items that measure the degree to which individuals desire and strive to achieve the bodies of athletes portrayed in the media (e.g., "I wished I looked as athletic as sports stars"). High internal consistency has been shown for the 4 dimensions in non-clinical (α = .96, .92, .95, and .96, respectively) and eating disordered populations (α = .94-.96, .94-.95, .93-.97, and .77-.84, respectively) as well as good construct validity (Calogero et al., 2004; Thompson et al., 2004). In the present study, the general and athletic internalization dimensions were combined for use in model testing given that the underlying construct of internalization is the same and to simplify interpretation of the data. Cronbach's alphas indicated high internal consistency for the information, pressures, and internalization dimensions examined in this study (α = .95, .96, and .86, respectively).

Drive for Thinness Subscale. The Eating Disorder Inventory—Drive for Thinness subscale (EDI—DT; Garner, 1991) assesses excessive concern with dieting, fear of weight gain, and preoccupation with a desire to be thinner. Excellent reliability and validity has been demonstrated in samples of eating disordered patients (Garner, 1991; Garner, Olmstead, & Polivy, 1983). In the present study, Cronbach's alpha indicated high internal consistency (α = .94).

Procedure

Women were administered the packet of questionnaires in counterbalanced order on admission to residential treatment. All of the assessment information was administered and collected in a sealed packet to maintain patient confidentiality. Informed consent was obtained prior to completion of any questionnaires.

RESULTS

Means, standard deviations, and the range of scores for self-objectification, body shame, dimensions of media influence, and drive for thinness are shown in Table I. The zero-order correlations among them are displayed in Table II.

TABLE I   Means and Variability for Measures at Admission to Treatment

Measure	M (SD)	Minimum	Maximum
Self-objectification	9.05 (13.53)	−25.00	25.00
Body shame	63.94 (19.77)	23.00	90.00
Drive for thinness	24.08 (12.42)	0.00	42.00
Media influence			
Information	29.90 (9.20)	9.00	45.00
Pressures	26.15 (7.70)	7.00	35.00
Internalization—general[a]	34.48 (9.26)	9.00	45.00
Internalization—athlete	18.36 (4.07)	5.00	25.00

NOTE: n = 209.
[a]Internalization—general and athlete were combined to produce one internalization score prior to model testing.

TABLE II   Correlations Among Measures

Measure	BS	Info	Press	Int-G	Int-A	DT
SO	.32	.29	.34	.49	.35	.38
BS	—	.28	.28	.36	.39	.44
Info	—	—	.55	.55	.41	.17
Press	—	—	—	.78	.48	.28
Int-G	—	—	—	—	.66	.38
Int-A	—	—	—	—	—	.39

NOTE: All correlations are significant at p < .01 except information/drive for thinness (ns). n = 209; SO = self-objectification; BS = body shame; Info = information; Press = pressures; Int-G = internalization—general; Int-A = internalization—athlete; DT = drive for thinness.

The Information dimension of the SATAQ-3 was the only variable not significantly correlated with drive for thinness. Positive correlations among self-objectification, body shame, and drive for thinness replicate previous findings with nonclinical samples (Fredrickson et al., 1998; Noll & Fredrickson, 1998). The mean self-objectification score in the current sample should be noted. Compared to nonclinical samples, the current mean self-objectification score of 9.05 is remarkably higher than the mean self-objectification scores previously reported, which have ranged between −10.34 and 7.70 (e.g., Fredrickson et al., 1998; Noll & Fredrickson, 1998; Tiggeman & Lynch, 2001; Tiggemann & Slater, 001).

Media Influence and Self-Objectification.   To test the relationship between media influence and self-objectification, the three dimensions of media influence measured by the SATAQ-3 were entered hierarchically into a regression model with information first, pressures second, and internalization third, based on their theoretical temporal order. When self-objectification was regressed on the SATAQ-3, Information, $\beta = .08$, t(206) $= 1.09$, p $= .28$, and Pressures, $\beta = -.003$, t(206) $= -0.03$, p $= .24$, from media were not significant predictors of self-objectification. Internalization of media was the only significant predictor; it accounted for 8% of the variance in self-objectification, $\beta = .41$, t(206) $= 4.56$, p $< .0001$, and the entire model explained 21% of the variance, F(3, 206) $= 17.14$, p $< .0001$.

Media Influence, Self-Objectification, and Drive for Thinness. The two mediational models of eating disorder pathology were tested using multiple regression analyses. According to Baron and Kenny (1986), 3 steps are necessary to establish mediation. In the first step, the predictor variable must correlate with the outcome variable. In the second step, the predictor variable must correlate with the hypothesized mediator. In the third step, when the predictor and mediator are entered simultaneously into the regression equation, the mediator must correlate with the outcome variable and the relationship between the predictor and the outcome should weaken.

Because internalization was the only significant predictor of self-objectification, it was the only factor of the SATAQ-3 included in the test of the first mediational model. Figure 1 [figure deleted] displays the results of a series of regression equations computed to test this model. In the first equation, internalization was a significant predictor of drive for thinness; it accounted for 15% of the variance, $\beta = .38$, t $= 4.63$, p $< .0001$. In the second equation, internalization was a significant predictor of self-objectification; it accounted for 24% of the variance, $\beta = .49$, t $= 7.90$, p $< .0001$. In the third equation, the amount of variance accounted for by internalization reduced from 15% to 8%, and self-objectification accounted for 5% of the variance independently. Overall, this mediational model accounted for 22% of the variance in drive for thinness, F(2,207) $= 15.62$, p $< .0001$. Thus, self-objectification partially mediated the relationship between internalization and drive for thinness, and internalization continued to contribute unique variance.

Self-Objectification, Body Shame, and Drive for Thinness. In the second analysis, a mediational model of eating disorders pathology was tested with self-objectification, body shame, and drive for thinness. In the first equation, self-objectification was a significant predictor of drive for thinness; it accounted for 14% of the variance, $\beta = .38$, t $= 4.39$, p $< .0001$. In the second equation, self-objectification was a significant predictor of body shame; it accounted for 10% of the variance, $\beta = .32$, t $= 4.87$, p $< .0001$. In the third equation, the amount of variance accounted for by self-objectification reduced from 14% to 7%, whereas body shame accounted for 17% of the variance. Overall, the mediational model accounted for 30% of the variance in drive for thinness, F(2,207) $= 23.89$, p $< .0001$. Thus, body shame partially mediated the relationship between self-objectification and drive for thinness in women with eating disorders, and self-objectification continued to contribute unique variance.

DISCUSSION

The present effort contributes to objectification theory by providing empirical evidence for the link between self-objectification and drive for thinness in a clinical sample of women with eating disorders. First, internalized media ideals for appearance, but not information or pressures from media about appearance, contributed to self-objectification. This suggests that the viewing of sexually objectifying images of women in visual media (e.g., magazines, music videos, television shows) may be a contributing factor to the chronic viewing of oneself as a sexual object if those images become integrated into one's self-perception. The informational and pressuring aspects of the media have a minimal effect on further self-objectification once media messages have been made part of an individual's own belief system.

This finding has implications for the exposure to and experience of media by children and adolescents. Due to the correlational nature of the data, the causal relationship among these variables is unclear. It could be that internalized media ideals are contributing to a self-objectified perspective of the self. In this case, media literacy programs in which individuals are taught to evaluate a wide variety of media critically may significantly diminish current and future self-objectification (Steiner-Adair & Vorenburg, 1999). However, it is possible that a self-objectified perspective on the self contributes to seeking out and internalizing media ideals for appearance. This perspective does not take as a given that, compared to men, women are just more susceptible to persuasion in advertising, and therefore more easily internalize media messages (see review, Martin, Gentry, & Hill, 1999). Rather, this possibility raises the question: Why do adolescent girls and women appear to be motivated to use the media for the purposes of social, emotional, and physical identity? It also requires researchers to move beyond appearance concerns in their measurements of and explanations for internalizing media and the experience of self-objectification to avoid cyclical theoretical reasoning for these phenomena.

Second, internalized media ideals predicted drive for thinness directly, and also indirectly, through self-objectification. This mediational model suggests that in women with eating disorders, internalized media ideals for appearance may lead to a drive for thinness without necessarily requiring the experience of self-objectification. However, the model with self-objectification explained slightly more variance, which suggests that it does contribute to the development and/or maintenance of the drive for thinness in women with eating disorders. These results support the theoretical assumptions that visual media encourage women to objectify themselves and that both internalized media ideals and self-objectification offer some account for eating disorders pathology.

Third, self-objectification predicted drive for thinness directly, and also indirectly, through body shame. This mediational model suggests that in women with eating disorders, self-objectification may lead to a drive for thinness without necessarily requiring the experience of body shame, which replicates previous tests of objectification theory in nonclinical samples (e.g., Fredrickson et al., 1998). However, the model with body shame explained substantially more variance, which suggests that it plays a significant role in the development and/or maintenance of a drive for thinness in women with eating disorders. The correlational nature of these two mediational models cannot establish conclusively the direction of effect, and thus causal links among these variables should be considered with caution. In sum, these findings suggest that self-objectification is present in women with eating disorders at admission to treatment; it negatively influences their emotional experiences, and it motivates the women to strive toward the attainment of unrealistic cultural body ideals.

As the length of hospitalization for women with eating disorders has significantly decreased over the past 15 years, it has become extremely important for inpatient programs to invest their time and energy optimally (Wiseman, Sunday, Klapper, Harris, & Halmi, 2001). Treatment programs may further benefit patients when they are in a severe stage of their eating disorder (i.e., when they require inpatient treatment) by including opportunities to address the experience of sexual and self-objectification in women's lives. Because women are socialized to experience their efforts to monitor and improve their physical appearance as self-chosen or "natural," this way of relating to the self may not be experienced as egodystonic, uncomfortable, or unpleasant (Costanzo, 1992; Johnston, 1997). Consequently, most women who enter treatment are unlikely to identify self-objectification as a problem because they are unaware that it is a potentially harmful, socially constructed form of self-perception. Certainly issues such as eating patterns, family dynamics, and individual psychological issues represent necessary therapeutic work. However, progress made in any of these areas may be undermined if socially constructed self-perceptions are not also targeted for change. When women continue to view themselves from a third person, rather than a first person, perspective, factors that contribute significantly to eating disorders pathology remain untouched.

In order to increase our understanding of the relationship between this kind of self-perception and recovery from eating disorders, further researchers should examine if and how self-objectification changes during treatment, and its specific effects on treatment outcomes including weight gain, symptomatic behavior, negative body image, self-esteem, interpersonal functioning, and time to relapse. In turn, this should point the way toward the development of treatment protocols for self-objectification and media literacy in both inpatient and outpatient settings. Prevention programs may further benefit from identifying and targeting the connections between self-perception, sociocultural influences, and eating behavior (e.g., GO GIRLS, 1999; Kater, 1998; Levine, Piran, & Stoddard, 1999).

It is important to note that the results of the present study are constrained by the operational definitions underlying the questionnaires administered and the self-report nature of the data. Although the questionnaires utilized here have been well validated, other measures may be more appropriate to assess the experiences under investigation. In the present effort, Noll and Fredrickson's (1998) SOQ was utilized in order to compare the scores of this clinical sample to previously tested nonclinical samples. Also, this was the same measure of self-objectification used initially to test propositions of objectification theory.

Roberts (2004) provided a recent comparison of McKinley and Hyde's (1996) Objectified Body Consciousness (OBC)-Surveillance subscale to the SOQ. This comparison demonstrated that the SOQ specifically captures the experience of viewing the body from an outsider's perspective whereas the OBC-Surveillance subscale includes items related to worry and concern about how the body appears to others. Thus, in the present sample of women who are particularly preoccupied with the body's outward appearance, the SOQ was considered an appropriate measure of this chronic, self-monitoring perspective of the self. However, the rank-order format of the scale has limitations, and one alternative measure of self-objectification for future research is McKinley and Hyde's (1996) OBC-Surveillance scale.

The measure of eating disorder pathology was also narrow and limited to one subscale of the EDI-2. Drive for thinness was used to capture the motivation for self-starvation in this population of women. Replication and/or efforts to extend this line of research might benefit from utilizing additional subscales of the EDI-2 or the Eating Disorders Examination (EDE; Fairburn & Wilson, 1993), as well as nonappearance and nonweight focused measures.

Katzman and Lee (1997) asserted that "one cannot affect individual elective starvation without somehow treating the social world these individuals inhabit" (p. 392). Because many Western cultures sexually objectify the female body, all women to varying degrees are vulnerable to the experiences of self-objectification and disordered eating. It is imperative that we challenge these experiences at a social and cultural level and that we educate women about the negative consequences of self-objectification early on in their physical, social, and emotional development. If children and adolescents can develop an empowered sense of self, they may be more likely to challenge power imbalances and the social construction of gender in ways that do not involve starvation and other abuses of their bodies (Katzman, Wooley, & Fallon, 1994). Overall, the results of the present study suggest that socio-cultural explanations for the development and maintenance of eating disorder pathology should continue to be explored and integrated into the prevention and treatment efforts for clinical and nonclinical populations of women.

REFERENCES

American Psychiatric Association. (1994). *Diagnostic and statistical manual of mental disorders* (4th ed.). Washington, DC: Author.

Baron, R. M., & Kenny, D. A. (1986). The moderator-mediator variable distinction in social psychological research: Conceptual, strategic, and statistical considerations. *Journal of Personality and Social Psychology, 51,* 1173–1182.

Bartky, S. L. (1990). *Femininity and domination: Studies in the phenomenology of oppression.* New York: Routledge.

Bruch, H. (1973). *Eating disorders: Obesity, anorexia nervosa, and the person within.* New York: Basic Books.

Bruch, H. (1982). Anorexia nervosa: Therapy and theory. *American Journal of Psychiatry, 139,* 1531–1538.

Calogero, R. M. (2004). A test of objectification theory: The effect of the male gaze on appearance concerns in college women. *Psychology of Women Quarterly, 28,* 16–21.

Calogero, R. M., Davis, W. N., & Thompson, J. K. (2004). The sociocultural attitudes toward appearance questionnaire (SATAQ-3): Reliability and normative comparisons of eating disordered patients. *Body Image, 1,* 193–198.

Costanzo, P. R. (1992). External socialization and the development of adaptive individuation and social connection. In D. N. Ruble, P. R. Costanzo, & M. E. Oliveri (Eds.), *The social psychology of mental health* (pp. 55–80). New York: Guilford.

Fairburn, C. G., & Wilson, G. T. (1993). *Binge eating: Nature, assessment, and treatment.* New York: Guilford Press.

Fredrickson, B. L., & Roberts, T. (1997). Objectification theory: Toward understanding women's lived experiences and mental health risks. *Psychology of Women Quarterly, 21,* 173–206.

Fredrickson, B. L., Roberts, T.-A., Noll, S. M., Quinn, D. M., & Twenge, J. M. (1998). That swimsuit becomes you: Sex differences in self-objectification, restrained eating, and math performance. *Journal of Personality and Social Psychology, 75,* 269–284.

Garner, D. M. (1991). *EDI-2: Eating disorder inventory professional manual.* Odessa, FL: Psychological Assessment Resources.

Garner, D. M., Olmstead, M. A., & Polivy, J. (1983). Development and validation of a multidimensional eating disorder inventory for anorexia nervosa and bulimia. *International Journal of Eating Disorders, 2,* 15–34.

GO GIRLS: *A curriculum for high school girls.* (1999). Seattle, WA: Eating Disorders Awareness and Prevention.

Groesz, L. M., Levine, M. P., & Murnen, S. K. (2002). The effect of experimental presentation of thin media images on body image satisfaction: A meta-analytic review. International *Journal of Eating Disorders, 31,* 1–16.

Johnston, J. (1997). Appearance obsession: Women's reactions to men's objectification of their bodies. In R. Levant & G. Brooks (Eds.), *Men and sex: New psychological perspectives* (pp. 61–83). New York: Wiley.

Kaschak, E. (1992). Engendered lives: A new psychology of women's experience. New York: Basic Books.

Kater, K. J. (1998). *Healthy body image: Teaching kids to eat and love their bodies too!* Seattle, WA: Eating Disorders Awareness and Prevention.

Katzman, M. A., & Lee, S. (1997). Beyond body image: The integration of feminist transcultural theories in the understanding of self-starvation. *International Journal of Eating Disorders, 22,* 385–394.

Katzman, M. A., Wooley, S. C., & Fallon, P. (1994). Eating disorders: A gendered disorder. *Eating Disorders Review, 5,* 1–3.

Kim, J. L., & Ward, L. M. (2004). Pleasure reading: Associations between young women's sexual attitudes and their reading of contemporary women's magazines. *Psychology of Women Quarterly, 28,* 48–58.

Levine, M. P., Piran, N., & Stoddard, C. (1999). Mission more probable: Media literacy, activism, and advocacy as primary prevention. In N. Piran, M. P. Levine, & C. Steiner-Adair (Eds.), *Preventing eating disorders: A handbook of interventions and special challenges* (pp. 3–25). Philadelphia: Brunner/Mazel.

Martin, M. C., Gentry, J. W., & Hill, R. P. (1999). The beauty myth and the persuasiveness of advertising: A look at adolescent girls and boys. In C. M. Macklin & L. Carlson (Eds.), *Advertising to children: Concepts and controversies* (pp. 165–187). Thousand Oaks, CA: Sage Publications.

McKinley, N. M., & Hyde, J. S. (1996). The objectified body consciousness scale. *Psychology of Women Quarterly, 20,* 181–215.

Noll, S. M., & Fredrickson, B. L. (1998). A mediational model linking self-objectification, body shame, and disordered eating. *Psychology of Women Quarterly, 22,* 623–636.

Roberts, T.-A. (2004). Female trouble: The menstrual self-evaluation scale and women's self-objectification. *Psychology of Women Quarterly, 28,* 22–26.

Slater, A., & Tiggemann, M. (2002). A test of objectification theory in adolescent girls. *Sex Roles, 46,* 343–349.

Steiner-Adair, C., & Vorenburg, A. P. (1999). Resisting weightism: Media literacy for elementary-school children. In N. Piran, M. P. Levine, & C. Steiner-Adair (Eds.), *Preventing eating disorders: A handbook of interventions and special challenges* (pp. 105–121). Philadelphia: Brunner/Mazel.

Stice, E. (2001). Risk factors for eating disorder pathology: Recent advances and future directions. In R. H. Striegel-Moore & L. Smolak (Eds.), *Eating disorders: Innovative directions in research and practice* (pp. 51–73). Washington, DC: American Psychological Association.

Thompson, J. K., van den Berg, P., Roehrig, M., Guarda, A. S., & Heinberg, L. J. (2004). The sociocultural attitudes toward appearance scale-3 (SATAQ-3): Development and validation. *International Journal of Eating Disorders, 35,* 293–304.

Tiggeman, M., & Lynch, J. (2001). Body image across the life span in adult women: The role of self-objectification. *Developmental Psychology, 37,* 243–253.

Tiggemann, M., & Slater, A. (2001). A test of objectification theory in former dancers and non-dancers. *Psychology of Women Quarterly, 25,* 57–64.

Wiseman, C. V., Sunday, S. R., Klapper, F., Harris, W. A., & Halmi, K. A. (2001). Changing patterns of hospitalization in eating disorder patients. *International Journal of Eating Disorders, 30,* 69–74.

DISCUSSION QUESTIONS

1. What is self-objectification?
2. What are some of the negative consequences of engaging in self-objectification?
3. What factor did the authors find led to or contributed to self-objectification in this study?
4. What are the implications of this study for treatment of women with eating disorders?

15

The Relationship Between Exercise Motives and Psychological Well-Being

John Maltby and Liza Day

ABSTRACT

The aim of the present study was to use the self-determination model of exercise motives to examine the relationship between extrinsic and intrinsic motives for exercise and a number of measures of psychological well-being. Undergraduate students purporting to exercise regularly (N = 227; 102 men, 125 women) were split into 2 groups: those exercising for less than 6 months and those exercising for 6 months or more. The respondents were asked to complete measures of exercise motivation, self-esteem, psychological well-being, and stress. Among individuals exercising for less than 6 months, a number of extrinsic motivations for exercise were significantly related to poorer psychological well-being. Among individuals exercising for 6 months or more, a number of intrinsic motivations were significantly related to better psychological well-being. The present findings suggest that researchers can use self-determination theory to understand the relationship between exercise motivation and psychological well-being.

The Journal of Psychology, Nov 2001 v135 i6 p651(10)
"The Relationship Between Exercise Motives and Psychological Well-Being (Statistical Data Included)" by John Maltby and Liza Day. © 2001 Heldref Publications

INTRODUCTION

Markland and Indledew (1997) introduced an improved measure of exercise motivation, Exercise Motivations Inventory 2 (EMI-2), to furnish additional theoretical propositions that distinguish between intrinsic and extrinsic motives for exercise. The EMI-2 contains 14 subscales and provides a comprehensive measure of exercise motivation; it focuses on internal (revitalization, enjoyment) and external (appearance) motivations. However, Markland and Ingledew argued that the scale reflects less conventional aspects of exercise motivation (e.g., social recognition) that relate to both internal and external aspects of exercise motives. Markland and Ingledew used Deci and Ryan's (1985, 1990) self-determination theory to extend the view that exercise may sometimes represent behavioral regulation. Within this perspective, individuals who have extrinsic reasons for beginning to exercise may eventually develop intrinsic motivations to exercise over time because their motives have become internalized.

The benefits of exercise to psychological well-being have been well documented. In particular, exercise is thought to reduce depression (Bybee, Zigler, Berliner, & Merisca, 1996; Craft & Landers, 1998; Rief & Hermanutz, 1996; Steptoe, Lipsey, & Wardle, 1998) and stress (Bundy, Carroll, Wallace, & Nagle, 1998; Kerr & Vanden Wollenberg, 1997; Rodgers & Gauvin, 1998; Steptoe et al., 1998; Stetson, Rahn, Dubbert, Wilner, & Mercury, 1997) and to heighten self-esteem (Asci, Kin, & Kosar, 1998; DuCharme, Bray, & Brawley, 1998; Loland, 1998; Rodgers & Gauvin, 1998) and general health (Daley & Parfitt, 1996; Szabo, Mesko, Caputo, & Gill, 1998). Furthermore, some authors have argued that there is a significant relationship between exercise motives and psychological well-being. Extrinsic motives for exercise are thought to lead to stress in individuals, whereas intrinsic motives for exercise are thought to lead to a release of stress (Bakker, Whiting, & van der Brug, 1997; Markland & Ingledew, 1997). Causal relationships between feelings of stress and poorer psychological well-being and between the release of stress and better psychological well-being suggest a relationship between exercise motives and psychological well-being—that is, that extrinsic motivations for exercise will result in poorer psychological well-being and intrinsic motivations for exercise will lead to better psychological well-being (Markland & Ingledew, 1997).

Within self-determination theory, the motivation to exercise is thought to alter over time, suggesting that the relationships between exercise motives and their correlates, such as psychological well-being, may be best considered over time. However, at present, there are no data that enable researchers to combine the recently developed EMI-2 (which is thought to reflect aspects of self-determination theory) and self-determination theory to examine the relationship between exercise motivations and psychological well-being. More specifically, exercise motivations are thought to change over time. Therefore, the benefits to psychological well-being of intrinsic exercise motives may only become apparent among those individuals who have been exercising for a long period of time.

Similarly, the relationship between extrinsic motives for exercise and poorer psychological well-being will be most apparent in individuals who have been exercising for a shorter period of time. Therefore, one can predict that, in the short-term, extrinsic exercise motives will be accompanied by poorer psychological well-being, whereas in the longer term, intrinsic exercise motives will be accompanied by better psychological well-being. Our aim in the present study was to examine the self-determination model and its predicted relationship with psychological well-being by comparing extrinsic and intrinsic motives with measures of psychological well-being, making the distinction between individuals exercising for shorter and longer periods of time.

METHOD

Participants

Five hundred fifty-six undergraduate students (252 men, 304 women), ages 18–42 (M = 28.3, SD = 5.3) responded to the survey. Consistent with Markland and Ingledew (1997), we included only those respondents who purported to exercise regularly (N = 227; 102 men, 125 women). Regular exercise was defined as exercising (e.g., swimming, jogging, weight training, aerobics) at least two to three times per week or participating in sports (e.g., golf, hockey, football) at least two to three times per week. A preliminary item on the survey asked the participants how many years and months they had been exercising regularly up to the present day. In further concordance with Markland and Ingewood (1997), a median split of two subsamples was formed; the first comprised individuals exercising for less than 6 months (n = 102), and the second comprised individuals exercising for 6 months or longer (n = 125).

Questionnaires

The respondents were asked to complete four questionnaires. The EMI-2 (Markland & Ingledew, 1997) includes 51 items measuring 14 motives for exercising: Stress Management, Revitalization, Enjoyment, Challenge, Social Recognition, Affiliation, Competition, Health Pressures, Ill-Health Avoidance, Positive Health, Weight Management, Appearance, Strength & Endurance, and Nimbleness. Each of the scales from the EMI-2 demonstrates good internal reliability, ranging from .69 to .95, and there is strong support for the factorial validity of the instrument and invariance of the factor structure across gender (Markland, in press; Markland & Ingledew, 1997).

The 12-item general Self-Esteem subscale of the Self-Description Questionnaire III (SDQIII; Marsh, 1990) was modified from the original

Rosenberg Self-Esteem Scale (Rosenberg, 1965). Both the manual for the SDQIII (Marsh, 1990) and two reports on the reliability and validity of the scale (Hunter & Stringer, 1993; Maltby, 1995) suggest confidence for using the scale with the present sample. Higher scores on this variable indicate a higher level of self-esteem.

We also used the 28-item version of the General Health Questionnaire (Goldberg & Williams, 1991). Factor analytic examination of the items within the General Health Questionnaire suggested four subscales: Somatic Symptoms, Anxiety/Insomnia, Social Dysfunction, and Severe Depression. Higher scores on each of these subscales indicate poorer psychological well-being on each of these traits.

The Hassles Scale contained within the Hassles and Uplifts Scales (Lazarus & Folkman, 1989) measures eight different aspects of stress. The scales were devised from a factor analysis of hassle statements rated within a particular time frame (either the past month, past week, yesterday, today, or other) and suggest hassles surrounding Future Security, Time Pressures, Work, Household Responsibilities, Health, Inner Concerns, Financial Responsibilities, and Neighborhood and Environment. For the present study, the respondents were asked to rate hassles within the time frame of the past week.

RESULTS

Satisfactory internal reliability statistics (Cronbach, 1951) above a = .71 were found for all the scales. These findings are consistent with the psychometric properties reported by the respective scales' authors (Goldberg & Williams, 1991; Lazarus & Folkman, 1989; Markland & Ingledew, 1997; Marsh, 1990). Table 1 contains the mean and standard deviation scores on each of the subscales of the EMI-2 by individuals exercising for less than 6 months and individuals exercising for 6 months or more.

Those individuals exercising for more than 6 months scored significantly higher on Stress Management, Enjoyment, and Challenge exercise motives than those exercising for less than 6 months. Furthermore, those individuals exercising for less than 6 months scored significantly higher on Social Recognition, Affiliation, and Competition exercise motives than those exercising for 6 months or more. These differences are consistent with the view that exercise motives change over time and that persons exercising for longer periods of time will demonstrate intrinsic (stress management, enjoyment, and challenge) rather than extrinsic (social recognition, affiliation, and competition) motives for exercising.

Because of these differences between intrinsic and extrinsic motives for exercising by period of time spent exercising, we computed Pearson product–moment correlation coefficients between exercise motives and psychological well-being, using the distinction between individuals exercising for

TABLE 1   Means and Standard Deviations for Scores on Each Subscale of the
Exercise Motivation Inventory 2, by Individuals Exercising < 6 Months
and ≥ 6 Months

Subscale	Exercising < 6 months n = 102		Exercising ≥ 6 months n = 125		
	M	SD	M	SD	t
Stress Management	2.20	1.5	2.94	1.2	−4.22 (*)
Revitalization	2.78	1.3	3.06	1.0	−1.87
Enjoyment	2.21	1.5	2.77	1.3	−3.06 (*)
Challenge	1.67	1.1	2.34	1.3	−4.11 (*)
Social Recognition	1.35	1.4	0.85	1.1	3.00 (*)
Affiliation	1.99	1.4	1.33	1.2	3.87 (*)
Competition	1.75	1.7	1.06	1.5	3.23 (*)
Health Pressures	1.23	1.4	0.98	1.4	1.58
Ill-Health Avoidance	2.87	1.3	2.89	1.4	−.13
Positive Health	3.57	1.3	3.53	1.3	.22
Weight Management	2.59	1.3	2.97	1.5	−1.88
Appearance	1.74	1.6	2.13	1.5	−1.88
Strength	2.59	1.4	2.67	1.3	−.41
Nimbleness	2.89	1.5	2.85	1.3	.20

(*)p < .01.

less than 6 months and those exercising for 6 months or more. Table 2 contains the Pearson product—moment correlations computed between the exercise motives measures and the Self-Esteem scale and subscales of the General Health Questionnaire. Pearson product—moment correlation coefficients were computed between the EMI-2 and the Hassles Scales. Table 3 contains the Pearson product–moment correlations that were computed between the exercise motives measures and the Time Pressures, Work, Health, and Inner Concerns subscales of the Hassles Index by those individuals exercising for less than 6 months and by those exercising for 6 months or more. No significant relationships were found between exercise motives and the remaining subscales of the Hassles Index (Future Security, Household Responsibilities, Financial Responsibilities, Neighborhood and Environment).

A number of significant correlations occurred between the exercise motives and psychological well-being measures. In comparing the subsamples (created by distinctions in length of exercise), we found a consistent pattern regarding a number of measures of exercise motives and the measures contained within the General Health Questionnaire and the Self-Esteem subscale of the SDQIII, which is consistent with the predictions expected within self-determination theory. Among the participants who had been exercising for less than 6 months, higher scores on extrinsic exercise motives (Social Recognition, Affiliation,

TABLE 2 Pearson Product-Moment Correlations Computed Between the Exercise Motives Measures and the Self-Esteem Scale, and the Subscales of the General Health Questionnaire for Individuals Exercising < 6 Months and Those Exercising ≥ 6 Months

Self-Esteem

Scale	< 6 Months (n = 102)	≥ 6 Months (n = 125)
Stress Management	−.20 (*)	.23 (**)
Revitalization	.02	.34 (**)
Enjoyment	.07	.26 (**)
Challenge	.11	.29 (**)
Social Recognition	−.33 (**)	.12
Affiliation	−.24 (**)	.15
Competition	−.26 (**)	.14
Health Pressures	−.32 (**)	.12
Ill-Health Avoidance	.04	.17 (*)
Positive Health	−.03	.34 (**)
Weight Management	−.28 (**)	.10
Appearance	−.26 (**)	.15
Nimbleness	.07	−.09

Somatic Symptoms

Scale	< 6 Months (n = 102)	≥ 6 Months (n = 125)
Stress Management	.23 (*)	−.30 (**)
Revitalization	−.07	−.28 (**)
Enjoyment	.15	−.31 (**)
Challenge	−.06	−.27 (**)
Social Recognition	.31 (**)	.01
Affiliation	.29 (**)	.02
Competition	.26 (**)	.01
Health Pressures	.22 (*)	−.08
Ill-Health Avoidance	.09	−.15
Positive Health	−.11	−.34 (**)
Weight Management	.15	−.08
Appearance	.28 (**)	−.13
Nimbleness	.10	.01

Anxiety, Insomnia

Scale	< 6 Months (n = 102)	≥ 6 Months (n = 125)
Stress Management	.34 (**)	−.26 (**)
Revitalization	−.01	−.34 (**)
Enjoyment	.10	−.35 (**)
Challenge	.08	−.24 (**)
Social Recognition	.32 (**)	.17 (*)
Affiliation	.26 (**)	.07
Competition	.24 (**)	.06

Continued

TABLE 2 *Continued*

Scale	< 6 Months (n = 102)	≥ 6 Months (n = 125)
Health Pressures	.28 (**)	−.15
Ill–Health Avoidance	−.15	−.16
Positive Health	.16	−.34 (**)
Weight Management	.22 (*)	−.06
Appearance	.26 (**)	−.30 (**)
Nimbleness	−.02	.14

Social Dysfunction

Scale	< 6 Months (n = 102)	≥ 6 Months (n = 125)
Stress Management	.22 (*)	−.20 (*)
Revitalization	.12	−.33 (**)
Enjoyment	.08	−.29 (**)
Challenge	.06	−.30 (**)
Social Recognition	.27 (**)	−.30 (**)
Affiliation	.33 (**)	.02
Competition	.24 (**)	.04
Health Pressures	.10	−.30 (**)
Ill–Health Avoidance	.08	−.23 (**)
Positive Health	.09	−.33 (**)
Weight Management	−.12	−.26 (**)
Appearance	.23 (*)	−.27 (**)
Nimbleness	−.01	.10

Severe Depression

Scale	< 6 Months (n = 102)	≥ 6 Months (n = 125)
Stress Management	.20 (*)	−.19 (*)
Revitalization	.02	−.26 (**)
Enjoyment	−.06	−.25 (**)
Challenge	−.03	−.25 (**)
Social Recognition	.28 (**)	.13
Affiliation	.34 (**)	−.02
Competition	.29 (**)	.04
Health Pressures	.27 (**)	−.15
Ill–Health Avoidance	−.01	−.28 (**)
Positive Health	.04	−.26 (**)
Weight Management	.05	−.11
Appearance	.21 (*)	−.12
Nimbleness	−.01	.04

(*) $p < .05$.
(**) $p < .01$.

TABLE 3 Pearson Product-Moment Correlations Computed Between the Exercise Motive Measures and the Time Pressures, Work, Health, and Inner Concerns Subscales of the Hassles Index by Individuals Exercising < 6 Months and Those Exercising ≥ 6 Months

Time Pressures

Scale	< 6 Months (n = 102)	≥ 6 Months (n = 125)
Stress Management	.31 (★★)	−.26 (★★)
Revitalization	−.10	−.33 (★★)
Enjoyment	.13	−.27 (★★)
Challenge	−.12	.12
Social Recognition	.33 (★★)	−.03
Affiliation	.31 (★★)	.05
Competition	.29 (★★)	−.10
Health Pressures	−.12	−.06
Ill-Health Avoidance	−.06	.08
Positive Health	.07	−.28 (★★)
Weight Management	.27 (★★)	−.21 (★)
Appearance	.23 (★)	.07
Nimbleness	.12	.15

Work

Scale	< 6 Months (n = 102)	≥ 6 Months (n = 125)
Stress Management	.15	−.31 (★★)
Revitalization	.07	−.39 (★★)
Enjoyment	.12	−.29 (★★)
Challenge	.11	.03
Social Recognition	.34 (★★)	−.06
Affiliation	−.12	−.11
Competition	.08	−.04
Health Pressures	.13	.12
Ill-Health Avoidance	.32 (★★)	−.13
Positive Health	.16	−.31 (★★)
Weight Management	.24 (★★)	−.03
Appearance	.04	.07
Nimbleness	−.15	.02

Health

Scale	< 6 Months (n = 102)	≥ 6 Months (n = 125)
Stress Management	.31 (★★)	−.35 (★★)
Revitalization	.30 (★★)	−.29 (★★)
Enjoyment	.26 (★★)	−.32 (★★)
Challenge	−.04	−.30 (★★)
Social Recognition	.31 (★★)	.02
Affiliation	.36 (★★)	−.01
Competition	.31 (★★)	.08

Continued

TABLE 3 *Continued*

Scale	< 6 Months (n = 102)	≥ 6 Months (n = 125)
Health Pressures	.49 (★★)	−.12
Ill-Health Avoidance	.26 (★★)	−.06
Positive Health	.33 (★★)	−.14
Weight Management	.30 (★★)	−.13
Appearance	−.03	.03
Nimbleness	.11	.02

Inner Concerns

Scale	< 6 Months (n = 102)	≥ 6 Months (n = 125)
Stress Management	.12	−.32 (★★)
Revitalization	.16	−.25 (★★)
Enjoyment	.04	−.27 (★★)
Challenge	−.01	.08
Social Recognition	−.13	.01
Affiliation	.29 (★★)	−.02
Competition	.27 (★★)	.12
Health Pressures	.25 (★★)	.08
Ill-Health Avoidance	.11	.11
Positive Health	.39 (★★)	−.11
Weight Management	.31 (★★)	−.14
Appearance	.22 (★)	.09
Nimbleness	.04	.01

(★) $p < .05$.
(★★) $P < .01$.

Competition, Appearance) were accompanied by higher scores on Somatic Symptoms, Anxiety, Social Dysfunction, Depression and lower scores on the Self-Esteem subscale. Furthermore, among the participants who had been exercising for 6 months or more, higher scores on some of the measures of intrinsic exercise motives (Revitalization, Enjoyment, Challenge) were accompanied by lower scores on Somatic Symptoms, Anxiety, Social Dysfunction, and Depression and higher scores on the Self-Esteem subscale.

The pattern of these correlations is partly replicated with some of the measures of stress. Among these correlations, higher levels of Time Pressure, Health, and Inner Concerns measures of the Hassles Scale shared a significant positive association with aspects of extrinsic exercise motives (Affiliation, Competition, Social Recognition) among those individuals exercising for less than 6 months. Furthermore, a significant negative correlation occurred between higher levels of Time Pressure, Health, and the Inner Concerns measures of the Hassles Scale and intrinsic exercise motives (Stress Management, Revitalization, Enjoyment) among those individuals exercising for 6 months or more.

DISCUSSION

The present findings suggest that, in the short term, extrinsic exercise motives for exercise are significantly related to poorer psychological well-being, whereas in the long term, intrinsic exercise motives for exercise are related to aspects of better psychological well-being. These findings are consistent with two theoretical standpoints. First, we found that extrinsic exercise motives are related to poorer psychological well-being, whereas intrinsic exercise motives for exercise are accompanied by better psychological well-being (Markland & Ingledew, 1997). Second, the present findings support Markland and Ingledew's suggestion that self-determination theory (Deci & Ryan, 1985, 1990) is crucial to understanding the relationship between exercise motivation and psychological well-being. That is, individuals' motivations for exercise change over time from extrinsic motives to more intrinsic motives.

Within this theory, one could argue that a dynamic process accounts for the shift from the significant relationship between extrinsic motivations and poorer psychological well-being to the significant relationship between intrinsic exercise motivations and better psychological well-being. This process would be consistent with the view that individuals internalize exercise motivation over time and that this affects psychological well-being. However, this interpretation assumes that this change over time is causal, with intrinsic exercise motives causing better psychological well-being. It is perhaps more likely that a more integrative relationship occurs whereby exercise motive and psychological well-being interact, through reinforcement of positive feelings, and exercise becomes more rewarding. Future researchers should expand on the present methodology and findings to examine this interaction, perhaps using longitudinal data.

Notwithstanding these speculations, the present findings suggest that one can use the combination of the concepts of self-determination theory and exercise motivations to examine the relationship between exercise motives and psychological well-being. Researchers should pursue this research area with confidence by using longitudinal data to gain further insight into relationships, over time, between exercise motives and psychological well-being.

REFERENCES

Asci, F. H., Kin, A., & Kosar, S. N. (1998). Effect of participation in an 8-week aerobic dance and step aerobics program on physical self-perception and body image satisfaction. *International Journal of Sport Psychology, 29,* 366–375.

Bakker, F. C., Whiting, H. T. A., & van der Brug, H. (1997). *Sport psychology: Concepts and applications.* London: Wiley.

Bundy, C., Carroll, D., Wallace, L., & Nagle, R. (1998). Stress management and exercise training in chronic stable angina pectoris. *Psychology and Health, 13,* 147–155.

Bybee, J., Zigler, E., Berliner, D., & Merisca, R. (1996). Guilt, guilt-evoking events, depression, and eating disorders. *Current Psychology, 15,* 113–127.

Craft, L. L., & Landers, D. M. (1998). The effect of exercise on clinical depression and depression resulting from mental illness: A meta-analysis. *Journal of Sport & Exercise Psychology, 20,* 339–357.

Cronbach, L. J. (1951). Coefficient alpha and the internal structure of tests. *Psychometrika, 16,* 297–334.

Daley, A. J., & Parfitt, G. (1996). Good health—Is it worth it? Mood states, physical wellbeing, job satisfaction and absenteeism in members and non-members of a British corporate health and fitness club. *Journal of Occupational and Organizational Psychology, 69,* 121–134.

Deci, E. L., & Ryan, R. M. (1985). *Intrinsic motivation and self-determination in human behavior.* New York: Plenum.

Deci, E. L., & Ryan, R. M. (1990). A motivational approach to self: Integration in personality. In R. A. Dienstbier (Ed.), Nebraska symposium on motivation: Vol. 38. *Perspectives on motivation* (pp. 237–288). Lincoln: University of Nebraska Press.

DuCharme, K. A., Bray, S. R., & Brawley, L. R. (1998). Predicting community exercise attendance using self-efficacy and goal cognitions. *Journal of Sport & Exercise Psychology, 20,* S22.

Goldberg, D., & Williams, P. (1991). *A user's guide to the general health questionnaire.* London: NFER Nelson.

Hunter, J. A., & Stringer, M. (1993). A short measure of self-esteem. Some data on reliability. *Perceptual and Motor Skills, 76,* 425–426.

Kerr, J. H., & Vanden Wollenberg, A. E. (1997). High and low intensity exercise and psychological mood states. *Psychology & Health, 12,* 603–618.

Lazarus, R. S., & Folkman, S. (1989). *Manual for the Hassles and Uplifts Scales.* Palo Alto, CA: Consulting Psychologists Press.

Loland, N. W. (1998). Body image and physical activity: A survey among Norwegian men and women. *International Journal of Sport Psychology, 29,* 339–365.

Maltby, J. (1995). A short measure of general self-esteem among Northern Irish university students: Some data on reliability. *Perceptual and Motor Skills, 81,* 1201–1202.

Markland, D. (2000). The Exercise Motivations Inventory-2. In J. Maltby, C. A. Lewis, & A. P. Hill (Eds.), *Commissioned reviews of 250 psychological tests* (pp. 58–60). Lampeter, Wales: Edwin Mellen Press.

Markland, D., & Ingledew, D. K. (1997). The measurement of exercise motives: Factorial validity and invariance across gender of a revised exercise motivations inventory. *British Journal of Health Psychology, 2,* 361–376.

Marsh, H. W. (1990). *Self-Description Questionnaire: SDQ III manual.* Campbelltown: University of Western Sydney, Macarthur.

Rief, W., & Hermanutz, M. (1996). Responses to activation and rest in patients with panic disorder and major depression. *British Journal of Clinical Psychology, 35,* 605–616.

Rodgers, W. M., & Gauvin, L. (1998). Heterogeneity of incentives for physical activity and self-efficacy in highly active and moderately active women exercisers. *Journal of Applied Social Psychology, 28,* 1016–1029.

Rosenberg, M. (1965). *Society and the adolescent self-image.* Princeton, NJ: Princeton University Press.

Steptoe, A., Lipsey, Z., & Wardle, J. (1998). Stress, hassles and variations in alcohol consumption, food choice and physical exercise: A diary study. *British Journal of Health Psychology, 3,* 51–63.

Stetson, B. A., Rahn, J. M., Dubbert, P. M., Wilner, B. I., & Mercury, M. G. (1997). Prospective evaluation of the effects of stress on exercise adherence in community-residing women. *Health Psychology, 16,* 515–520.

Szabo, A., Mesko, A., Caputo, A., & Gill, E. T. (1998). Examination of exercise-induced feeling states in four modes of exercise. *International Journal of Sport Psychology, 29,* 376–390.

DISCUSSION QUESTIONS

1. What are some examples of internal or intrinsic motivations for exercising? What area some examples of external or extrinsic motivations for exercising?

2. What are some of the benefits of exercise for psychological well-being?

3. What did the researchers find were some of the differences between people who had been exercising for more than 6 months and people who had been exercising for less than 6 months?

4. What do the authors find with respect to intrinsic and extrinsic motives for exercising and psychological well-being?

5. What are the implications of these findings for people who are about to begin an exercise program and want to stay committed to it in the long-term?

16

Ethical Issues Involved in the Role of Psychologists in Medical Settings

Geraldine Lucignano and Sandra Lee

ABSTRACT

Psychologists work in various medical settings, but there is no consensus as to their role in these settings. Role delineation, working within the medical model, multiple responsibilities, and confidentiality are all issues that need to be addressed in this context. Often, psychologists function as part of an interdisciplinary team, but even when they are looked to as providers of psychological services, similar services are provided by other team members as well. There is also pressure for the psychologist to adhere to the medical model, in which the physician is the implied leader of the team. To illustrate the difficulties psychologists face in medical settings, the example of patient noncompliance is appropriate. The psychologist views noncompliance not in terms of good-patient versus bad-patient behavior, but as a result of the influences on patient behavior that are experienced in the hospital environment. Noncompliance is not seen as symptomology by the psychologist, as many medical personnel label it. The psychologist must therefore work independently with the patient. Treatment planning in medical institutions is often accomplished by a treatment team approach, and the psychologist must consider the effects on the team, medical setting, and patient before making recommendations. The medical setting can be coercive, and the psychologist cannot be swayed by this. Confidentiality can be a problem as well because patient records, as a means of communication

The Journal of Rehabilitation, April-June 1991 v57 n2 p55(3)
"Ethical Issues Involved in the Role of Psychologists in Medical Settings" by Geraldine Lucignano and Sandra Lee. © 1991 National Rehabilitation Association

between staff members, are not under the direct supervision of psychologists; after docu-
mentation is made in a chart, the psychologist no longer has control over who sees the
information. It is essential that psychologists be included in hospital policy planning in
the future so that their ability to do their jobs is protected. This will take persistence and
political activism, but the end result will be improved status as a discipline within the
medical setting. (Consumer Summary produced by Reliance Medical Information, Inc.)
This paper identifies the specific ethical concerns related to the role and functioning of
psychologists in medical settings. Literature regarding role delineation, working within
the medical model, multiple responsibilities and confidentiality is addressed. Several
strategies are proposed for integrating psychological models in medical settings.

INTRODUCTION

Psychologists can be found working in various medical settings including general hospitals, physical rehabilitation centers, and chronic disease settings. It is estimated that over 10% of the American Psychological Association (APA) members work in medical settings, with an increase of 200 to 300 each year (DeLeon, Pallak & Heffernan, 1982). As this number continues to grow, there is an increasing need to focus on areas of ethical concern related to working in these settings. Important ethical concerns involve role delineation, working within the medical model, multiple responsibilities, and confidentiality.

Role Delineation

Role delineation is of primary ethical concern since it lays the ground work for the responsibilities and expectations of the psychologist. However, there is no consensus as to what constitutes the role of the psychologist in a medical setting (Schofield, 1976). Diverse terminology has been used to describe this role. These terms include health psychology, medical psychology, clinical psychology, and behavioral medicine (Korchin & Schuldberg, 1981; Wiggins, 1976). It is argued that this lack of clarity in definition of terms is more than semantic confusion. Asken states, ". . . (psychologists) can never be sure whether their interests and activities have or have not been included under one of these nonstandardized terms" (Asken, 1979, p. 66).

The psychologist in a medical setting often functions as part of a multidisciplinary team. This team usually includes a physician, social worker, speech pathologist, physical and occupational therapist. Although the team may view the psychologist as having a legitimate role, they may also condone the delivery of services of a psychological nature by other team members. This was demonstrated in a recent investigation of the psychologist's role in a physical rehabilitation setting (Remenyi, Thomas & Leonard, 1981). In this survey 111 team members were given questionnaires and asked to comment on role descriptions. The results indicated that the physician is viewed as the appropriate person to lead case conferences and to assess clients for brain damage, the occupational therapist to conduct group therapy and training sessions, and the social worker to counsel clients and families regarding their adjustment. In addition, the psychologist was identified as the most appropriate team member to perform the traditional duties of personality and intelligence assessment. The authors conclude that historical biases, customary practices, and perceived areas of expertise were reasons for these observations.

Working Within the Medical Model

Ethical awareness is essential when providing psychological treatment within the medical milieu. The hospital environment includes unique areas of stress which affect both the patients and treatment team members. For example, Kastenbaum describes the hospital setting as analogous to a Greek city-state with the fundamental similarities being, ". . . inequality among classes of people and the proliferation of regulations to govern everyday life" (Kastenbaum, 1982, p. 158). As a result of this unique hospital milieu, Kastenbaum believes that there is a lack of objective decision making. He states, ". . . certain classes of people earn their right to exist only by carrying out carefully specified instructions and tasks" (Kastenbaum, 1982, p. 158). Contributions to the problem include the stress of territorial team issues, issues of job burnout, outmoded methods of providing services, a constant budget crisis, administration's focus on public relations, and errors in professional judgment which are covered up (Kastenbaum, 1982). Continued conflict between the medical model and psychological appraisal can place pressure on the psychologist to adhere to the medical milieu. This is of particular concern when working on a team which includes a physician as leader. The traditional medical model implies that the physician is the "expert," the patient is seen as having "diseased organs" which can be repaired, and "good patients" are those who comply with hospital staff (Elfant, 1984). In contrast to this, the psychologist is ethically responsible to work autonomously, regards the patient as being influenced by a variety of sources (such as environmental stress) and noncompliance with hospital procedure is seen as separate from symptomology (Weitlieb & Budman, 1979). The literature shows consensus as to psychologists' objection to working on a team with a physician as absolute leader. Most psychologists object to, ". . . the notion that psychological services ought to be organized under the auspices and authority of physicians" (Hoffman, 1979, p. 571). That is, they object to being referred clients only when deemed appropriate by the physician. Psychologists prefer to have equally autonomy on the medical team. This includes having admitting rights and autonomy in writing orders for treatment of their patients.

Multiple Responsibilities

In working within medical settings, many times, treatment planning is accomplished through a treatment team approach. During treatment planning the psychologist must consider the influence effected on the team, medical setting, and patient. The psychologist has responsibilities to all of these parties. According to Monahan the priority of these responsibilities is, ". . . rarely the same across situations but may change with each intervention strategy and set of circumstances" (Monahan, 1980, p. 129). The psychologist in a medical setting is both an employee and healer. Therefore, in situations where obligations to an employer and patient are not consistent there can be a serious ethical dilemma.

The psychologist should understand the effect of multiple responsibilities in order to keep the best interest of the patient in mind. According to the APA psychologists should not be swayed by, ". . . personal, social, organizational, financial, or political situations and pressures that might lead to misuse of their influence" (American Psychological Association [APA], 1981b, p. 633). While the medical setting's coerciveness is subtle (Hoffman, 1979), there may be a focus on suppressing undesirable behavior of the patient (Flanagan & Liberman, 1982). For example, the institution may focus on the patient's compliance with traditional treatment and prefer that patients not "excite" other patients by becoming a model of noncompliance. In contrast, a patient may be reluctant to take the "good patient" or "sick patient" role. This resistance to comply with the "sick" role may be indicative of independence. In other words, a particular patient's acting out behaviour may be an indication of a good prognosis and improved long term adjustment (Hoffman, 1979).

Confidentiality

Another important ethical concern is that of confidentiality of documentation. Many times, psychologists are required to document all of their activities in a manner appropriate to hospital procedures (American Psychological Association [APA], 1981a). Limited awareness of confidentiality on the part of other hospital staff directly influences the management of this documentation.

Once psychological entries are made into the medical chart, the psychologist no longer has direct control over the information. Hospital staff may be unaware of the ethical implications involved in the confidentiality of psychological reports. This information can be exposed to a wide range of staff including administrators, clerks, technicians, statisticians, and others (Siegel, 1979). In addition, when the patient is discharged, the chart is frequently sent to the medical records department of the hospital. Requests for information are usually sent directly to that department. Psychological information can be forwarded to other professionals or institutions without the consent of the client or psychologist.

Strategies for the Future

In order for psychologists to adhere to an effective role delineation, it is essential that they be involved in hospital policy making organizations. These organizations are typically dominated by physicians. One example is the Joint Commission on Accreditation of Hospitals (JCAH) which forms policies which directly effect psychologists. For example, they suggest standards for referral and documentation. It has been stated that, ". . . organized medicine will never easily give up its hegemony over the delivery of health care services in the United States" (Zaro, Ginsberg, Batchelor & Pallak, 1982, p.1344). Nevertheless, psychologists have been persistent in their interactions with JCAH and have made slow progress in their attempts to gain equal status as a discipline (Zaro et al., 1982).

Education may help to alleviate frustrations encountered in understanding the medical milieu and its effect on ethical dilemmas. For example, some suggest that psychology students have some exposure to a medical setting during their academic training (Matthews & Avis, 1982; Spear & Schoepke, 1981). The medical team's understanding of the psychologist's multiple responsibilities may foster greater cooperation in dealing with areas of ethical concern. One method of increasing understanding is the formation of a multidisciplinary committee designed to promote professional awareness of treatment team issues. This committee could operate at the hospital, state, or national level.

One strategy for overcoming ethical concerns involved in confidentiality is specific labeling for psychological entries in medical records. Cameron and Shepei (1981) found that stamping the psychological information "confidential" was unsuccessful. However, they found other methods of identifying this information more effective. One of these methods was to stamp the documents with "Not to be Copied or Released." Another was to include a notation in the chart indicating that information would be released following an appropriate request made directly to the psychologist.

Finally, some inroads to political activism by psychologists have begun. In 1982 the Association of Medical School Professors of Psychology was established (Thompson, 1987). This association is one attempt to address ethical concerns, yet more needs to be done. Until the time when an organized multidisciplinary understanding of ethical issues can be achieved, psychologists working in medical settings must continue to stand firm in upholding their standards regardless of pressure to do otherwise.

REFERENCES

American Psychological Association. (1981a). *Specialty guidelines for the delivery of services.* Washington, D.C.: Author.

American Psychological Association. (1981b). Ethical principles of psychologists. *American Psychologist. 36* (6), 633–638.

Asken, M. (1979). Medical psychology: Toward a definition. *Professional Psychology. 10,* 66–73.

Cameron, R., & Shepel, L. (Eds.). (1981). Strategies for preserving the confidentiality of psychological reports. *Canadian Psychology. 22* (2), 191–193.

DeLeon, P. H., Pallak, M.S., & Heffernan, J. A. (1982). Hospital health care delivery. *American Psychologist, 37* (12), 1340–1341.

Elfant, A. (1984). Psychotherapy and assessment in hospital settings: Ideological and professional conflicts. *Professional Psychology: Research and Practice, 16* (1), 55–63.

Flanagan, S. G., & Liberman, R. P. (1982). Ethical issues in the practice of behaviour therapy. In M. Rosenbaum (Ed.), *Ethics and values in psychotherapy: A guidebook* (pp. 207–237). New York: The Free Press.

Hoffman, I. (1979). Psychological versus medical psychotherapy. *Professional Psychology. 10,* 571–579.

Kastenbaum, R. (1982). The psychologist and hospital policy: A report from the real world. *American Psychologist, 12,* 1356–1359.

Korchin, S. J., & Schuldberg, D. (1981). The future of clinical assessment. *American Psychologist, 36* (10), 1147–1158.

Matthews, K. A., & Avis, N. E. (1982). Psychologists in schools of public health. Current status, future prospects, and implications for other health settings. *American Psychologist, 37,* 949–954.

Monahan, J. (1980). *Who is the client? The ethics of psychological intervention in the criminal justice system.* Washington, D.C.: American Psychological Association.

Remenyi, A. G., Thomas, s. A., & Leonard, R. (1981). Psychological services in rehabilitation. *American Psychologist, 16* (3), 361–368.

Schofield, W. (1976). The psychologist as a health professional. *Professional Psychology. 7,* 5–8.

Siegel, M. (1979). Privacy, ethics, and confidentiality. *Professional Psychology. 10,* 248–249.

Spear, J., & Schoepke, J. (1981). Psychologists and rehabilitation: Mandates and current training practices. *Professional Psychology, 12* (5), 606–612.

Thompson, R. (1987). A call for medical school activism. *The APA Monitor, 18* (2), 9.

Weitlieb, S., & Budman, S. H. (1979). Dimensions of role conflicts for health care psychologists. *Professional Psychology, 10,* 640–644.

Wiggins, J. G. (1976). The psychologist as a health professional in the health maintenance organization. *Professional Psychology, 7,* 9–13.

Zaro, J. S., Ginsberg, M. R., Batchelor, W. F., Pallak, M.S. (1982). Psychology and JCAH: Reflections on a decade of struggle. *American Psychologist. 37* (12), 1342–1349.

DISCUSSION QUESTIONS

1. What are some ethical issues that psychologists working in the medical system face?
2. Why do the authors believe there is a conflict for the psychologist working within the medical model?
3. Why is it crucial that the psychologist understand the effect of multiple responsibilities in the medical setting?
4. What are some strategies for overcoming these ethical issues in the future?

InfoMarks: Make Your Mark

What Is an InfoMark?

It is a single-click return ticket to any page, any result, or any search from InfoTrac College Edition.

An InfoMark is a stable URL, linked to InfoTrac College Edition articles that you have selected. InfoMarks can be used like any other URL, but they're better because they're stable—they don't change. Using an InfoMark is like performing the search again whenever you follow the link, whether the result is a single article or a list of articles.

How Do InfoMarks Work?

If you can "copy and paste," you can use InfoMarks.

When you see the InfoMark icon on a result page, its URL can be copied and pasted into your electronic document—web page, word processing document, or email. Once InfoMarks are incorporated into a document, the results are persistent (the URLs will not change) and are dynamic.

Even though the saved search is used at different times by different users, an InfoMark always functions like a brand new search. Each time a saved search is executed, it accesses the latest updated information. That means subsequent InfoMark searches might yield additional or more up-to-date information than the original search with less time and effort.

Capabilities

InfoMarks are the perfect technology tool for creating:

- Virtual online readers
- Current awareness topic sites—links to periodical or newspaper sources
- Online/distance learning courses
- Bibliographies, reference lists
- Electronic journals and periodical directories
- Student assignments
- Hot topics

Advantages

- Select from over 15 million articles from more than 5,000 journals and periodicals
- Update article and search lists easily
- Articles are always full-text and include bibliographic information
- All articles can be viewed online, printed, or emailed
- Saves professors and students time
- Anyone with access to InfoTrac College Edition can use it
- No other online library database offers this functionality
- FREE!

How to Use InfoMarks

There are three ways to utilize InfoMarks—in HTML documents, Word documents, and Email

HTML Document

1. Open a new document in your HTML editor (Netscape Composer or FrontPage Express).
2. Open a new browser window and conduct your search in InfoTrac College Edition.
3. Highlight the URL of the results page or article that you would like to InfoMark.
4. Right-click the URL and click Copy. Now, switch back to your HTML document.
5. In your document, type in text that describes the InfoMarked item.
6. Highlight the text and click on Insert, then on Link in the upper bar menu.
7. Click in the link box, then press the "Ctrl" and "V" keys simultaneously and click OK. This will paste the URL in the box.
8. Save your document.

Word Document

1. Open a new Word document.
2. Open a new browser window and conduct your search in InfoTrac College Edition.
3. Check items you want to add to your Marked List.
4. Click on Mark List on the right menu bar.
5. Highlight the URL, right-click on it, and click Copy. Now, switch back to your Word document.
6. In your document, type in text that describes the InfoMarked item.
7. Highlight the text. Go to the upper bar menu and click on Insert, then on Hyperlink.

8. Click in the hyperlink box, then press the "Ctrl" and "V" keys simultaneously and click OK. This will paste the URL in the box.
9. Save your document.

Email

1. Open a new email window.
2. Open a new browser window and conduct your search in InfoTrac College Edition.
3. Highlight the URL of the results page or article that you would like to InfoMark.
4. Right-click the URL and click Copy. Now, switch back to your email window.
5. In the email window, press the "Ctrl" and "V" keys simultaneously. This will paste the URL into your email.
6. Send the email to the recipient. By clicking on the URL, he or she will be able to view the InfoMark.